Blessed Bey

From Childhood to Death and Back
IBSN: **978-0-578-26505-6**

Blessed beyond Belief

Table of Contents:	1
Forward	2
Dedication	3
About the Author	4
Chap. 1: The Early Years	5
Chap. 2: The Change	36
Chap. 3: The Ongoing Health Issues	59
Chap. 4: The Beginning of the Latter	88
Back Cover	113

Forward

A lot of people may question my choice of stories throughout this book. Stick around until the last pages you will find out why these are near and dear to my heart as written. My mother used to tell me that I was special, special enough to have two sets of parents. You see I was adopted. My birth mom realized that she could not care for me by herself and like many birth fathers, mine didn't stick around. From reading the papers of my mother's requests for placement, I saw she felt that my birth father was more concerned about himself than her and the baby they created. Looking back and counting my mom must have conceived me in late August or early September 1965. From what I can put together from the papers that I have, my mom was 17 when I was born on June 5, 1966. She had just celebrated her birthday the previous month. Facing many obstacles, such as trying to finish high school, raise a baby by herself and family turmoil, my birth Mother weighed all of her options and after a few months of struggling alone she contacted social services and started the adoption process. Right here is the second of my many blessings, the first being her decision to go the *hard sacrifice* of teenage motherhood. After coming to grips with knowing the fact that she wanted to give better than she could provide was my third blessing. I never met my birth mother but I hope to do so one day because I would love to say to her from the bottom of my heart:

Thank You

<u>Dedication</u>

I want to thank everyone that had a hand in shaping me into the person I am today. As I look back on my life I realize that I seemed to squeeze a lot of living into my first thirty-one years of life. If I had ten million years and five mouths I could never thank GOD enough.

About the Author

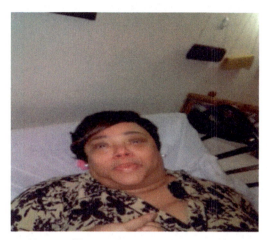

I'm Kimberly 55, a mom of three grown men and grandma to the best freshman football and basketball player, straight "A" puller of my heart's strings and a granddaughter I don't get to see often enough. I enjoy writing short stories and poetry.

At age thirty one, I had a car accident that left me paralyzed from my neck down The hospital and rehab can spoil you and lull you into a false sense of security After coming home to a new apartment I would look around first thing in the morning and before opening my eyes I would ask the Lord to make me normal or dead upon opening my eyes. After a few days I realized the incredible blessing I had been granted I changed that prayer into a thankful one. I then decided to live for my children. I knew I had to be the best mother I could despite my limitations. I still maintain a house, provided for the family, give loving guidance to the guys and supervise my own care. Being home just took on a new meaning. As time went on I realized things were slowly becoming our new normal and easier to navigate and dare I say comfortable.

One day I looked up and ten years had flown by. Each child has graduated high school. I also appreciated life more because I wasn't afraid to face the next challenge. I even rose to meet one; my counselor wanted me to participate in the Miss Wheelchair in 2009. I enjoyed that weekend but began having health issues and been bedridden dealing with skin problems ever since. Fast forwarding to today, I have learned how to take things in stride. I've found solace in writing. So **<u>Blessed beyond Belief</u>** was born out of my boredom, I hope you enjoy it!

Chapter 1 **The Early years**

Everyone's childhood memories run a gamut of emotions from love to crazy or a funny story or on the heels of a tragedy. Like the way mine, Kimberly Walker's new life began. My mother Barbara was a type 1 diabetic, diagnosed when she was 16 years old. My father often told me about how their marriage started on September 28, 1948 and my mother pulled a trifecta: they got married on Tuesday, she came down with measles by Monday the 4th, and was diagnosed with Diabetes by the 7th, that Thursday night. I once asked him if he knew that she was going to have so much baggage from the beginning would he have married her anyway… He replied with a huge smile on his face, "I've loved Little Red from the first time I saw her and I wouldn't take any of it back for any reason." If ever there was a man that loved a woman from the, top of her head to the bottom of her feet, it was my father Clem Thomas Walker, who was madly in love with Barbara Lee Arrington throughout their 35 year marriage. Seven years into their marriage my mom became pregnant. It was a difficult time from day one until she lost the baby in the sixth month. Back in that time no matter what happened to the baby the mother still had to give birth. My mother's health suffered both mentally and physically. She decided from that unfortunate loss that she never wanted to try to have another baby naturally. My dad told me that she became very depressed because of this. He was happy with their life together but my mother wanted a child. So in order to make Little Red happy, he wrapped his mind around the idea of adoption. They started the paperwork and counseling. The baby that they lost was a boy they named Warren. They attended one "Puppy Farm", the affectionate nickname my father gave the adoption warehouse. Although it's not "Daisy Hill" or "a baby warehouse", it is the only place you can see every child that is up for adoption at the same time. My father also told me that the morning of the visit to the puppy farm, he thought they had agreed on a little boy, but it seems I chose them. They were sitting on the couch in a room full of children of different ages, different sexes, and different colors. While they sat waiting for my social worker to join them, I crawled over and pulled up on my father's pants leg. My big brown eyes, and award-winning smile melted his heart. When he turned to talk to me I reached at his goatee, and it was a done deal. Later I found out that my mom was happier that they got a girl instead of a boy. I didn't get to go home with them exactly then, but two days later, I was onto my new life.

I have been told a lot of colorful stories about my life, when I came to live with the Walker's. I was already 2 years old but not yet walking. Although I seem to be in very good health, the puppy farm workers didn't take the time to teach individual children how to walk. My mom explained "they probably were not allowed to show very much affection because it would be hard to get detached. Any attachment to the group home staff could hinder the child from forming bonds with the adopting family. Which could render that child "unadoptable". This is how it was explained by my social worker. Just like any home placement, Maxine Carter made visits frequently. As my parents progressed through the system, she changed her visits to every six months. Ms. Carter often commented in her notes "that Kimberly is progressing and rapidly making the transition. Although I still have concerns because she is still not walking". There came a time that Mrs. Carter actually threatened to remove me from the home if they didn't stop carrying me everywhere and teach me how to walk. It was the Sunday night before a Monday home visit, and contrary to everyone's urgings I still had shown no interest in walking. My mom had actually been reduced to tears earlier in the day, because she was afraid that I was going to be taken away the next day. Just like we did every Sunday evening we were in the den watching Tom Jones' variety hour and Tom Jones started to sing "What's new Pussycat?" I crawled over to the television set, proceeded to stand up and give Tom Jones a kiss, turned toward my dad who was sitting on the floor in front of the couch. When he spread his arms and legs and called me *"Chap"*, I ran to him that was the beginning of me walking ever since. Needless to say my mom was very overjoyed. The next day she wrote Tom Jones and told him thank you for making my daughter walk. She explained the events of the previous evening to him in this letter. A couple of weeks later we received an autographed picture of Tom Jones in the mail, which I still own today.

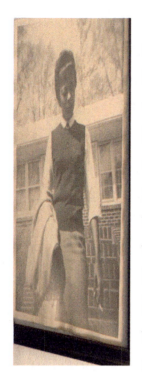 My aunt Peggy lived with us, she and my mother were inseparable. She had come to live with my mother while my dad was in the Army. For the first few years of their marriage my father was deployed. They were uncertain of whether the war would make a widow of my mom before her 21st birthday. The sisters used to dress like twins, even though they were ten years apart. One of my earliest memoriesmy aunt Peggy is that she used to work for a family around the corner from where my mom worked. We would drop her off on our way to my mom's job. They both worked from 8 to 12 as maids on Saturday mornings. After they got paid we would go shopping in Colonial Heights, Petersburg or Richmond Virginia. Every shopping trip we took on Saturdays my mom and my aunt would always buy me something. Spoiled much, a resoundingly YES!

It's an afternoon in June 1970, several days after my birthday; mom and I had just returned home from her job with Mrs. Pair. While mom is getting things out of the car, I start to ride my

Army car. This car is a steel frame pedal powered vehicle. Two days before I spotted one of the first Power Wheel cars ever made and just had to have it. Mommy told me if I was good the rest of the year that Santa Claus might bring it to me. There was no temper tantrum, or questioning the answer. Instead, I held the feelings inside until I got home. For anyone that knew my mother, you would say that I made the best choice. At five years old a child doesn't know how to express anger anyway except to cry, pout, or through a tantrum but these were none of the things that my mom would put up with. I learned this earlier in life, maybe a year or so back, in Woolworth's department store over a doll baby. I stood there with the doll baby in hand and cried for it. To add insult to injury when mommy told me to put it back I said *no*. With one fell swoop she grabbed the doll baby and put it back on the shelf, grabbed me and spanked my butt with her pocketbook strap. That was my first and only temper tantrum ever. It's amazing the learning curve. From that day forward I learned if I had feelings about anything that I should keep them to myself. Thus began my emotional wreckage.

Earlier that day while at the Pair's house, when it was time for me to eat lunch I didn't want what mom had brought with us. I just sat at the table picking at my food, not realizing that I was keeping mom from doing what she had to do. Being the underweight, finicky, anemic, sickly child that I was she took time out to have a tea party with me, just to get me to eat. Even though taking the time to do that made her late leaving and also cut her pay for the day. As a child we don't realize the great lengths a good mother goes to please the children, or to encourage them. At that time, mom didn't say much about my attitude, because Mrs. Pair was also in attendance at the tea party. After the luncheon I went to watch TV. Mom then had to double time it to finish work, because what I didn't know was that no matter how long it took for everything to be done she was still only going to be paid $10 for the day at that house and she still had to clean the mother-in-law's house located five miles away from our house in the county. Looking back now, as the saying goes "I may have cost more than I was worth sometimes". I'm glad my mother was willing to pay whatever price I cost. After we were in the car on the way home from senior Pair's place, that's when my mom expressed her disappointment in the way I had acted. Even though it was not still the 1940's, and Mrs. Pair was a progressive kind of white woman, I stepped way across that invisible line that remained ingrained in my mother's psyche. To her I'd basically said *I'm in charge of this lunch time and fall in your place or else.* Now that I'm an adult, I totally understand how it feels to "lose face", in front of your boss. To be shamed by your own child has got to be the worst. My mother was the "Queen of promises", although I was just fine with these promises, they were threats to spanking my butt. Today was once again such a promise, or so I thought, no sooner than she parked the car in the driveway, she grabbed the belt from around her waist and let me have it. Ten licks, maybe for the amount she was paid, or for the time it took to explain to her boss why she needed to take a break from cleaning the Silver she so hated doing every week. Nonetheless, whether it was punishment for my actions or her frustration, to her it was sanctioned. Too much was all I could think, but crying would make her stop I'm hoping every time the belt wrapped around my whole body. After she was done or tired out, which ever had occurred in her mind, she spun me around with tears in her eyes and said that famous phrase "this hurts me more than you"

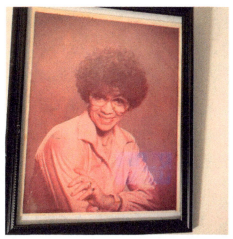 and kissed my cheek and said "go play". Standing there hurting too much to move, still crying, feeling rage for the first time, and wanting to explode; I couldn't figure out exactly what just happened. My usually mild mannered mother just turned into someone I didn't ever want to see again! Like every situation that involved anger for anyone, I looked for a place to unleash my rage. All I could think was ride it off. I slowly eased my still stinging bottom into my army car and pedaled as fast as my spindly little legs could move down the driveway as far as I was brave enough to go. Which was only to the turn to enter the yard from the long way around. Passing the apple trees, spotting two that had fallen that looked like they'd be tasty enough to bring back the joyful mom that I've grown so close to feeling safe with. Even though not knowing it then, acceptance is crucial to a child's survival. With a peace offering tucked in the trunk of my war machine, I raced back to the front yard with the same amount of vigor that I'd rode off with. So determined to right my wrong, I'm pedaling with my head down as if to

count every blade of grass that I saw pass beneath the opened floor. Racing so fast that I never saw the front of my brand new Power Wheel orange Corvette emerging from behind my mom's car until my dad yelled "STOP"! My mom tried to back up the Corvette but unfortunately I looked over at him and plowed into the side of it. I'm going so fast that the impact throws my army car rear end up in the air. I slipped in such a way that I'm thrown to my knees and hit my forehead on the steering wheel. Funny thing is, I went full circle in about ten or fifteen minutes. I left that very spot crying just to return to cry for a different reason. Although pain brought on both episodes, another lesson was learned, there's different kinds of pain.

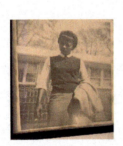

Aunt Peggy would try to hide any gift she purchased until we returned home and my mother would get mad with my aunt for spoiling me rotten. Aunt Peggy would use me as her gopher and I loved it. She was a salt-aholic and even though I was a picky eater every snack my aunt offered I would gobble it up and spoil my real meal, this seemed to make my mom jealous. Aunt Peggy lived with us until I was five. I told my mom that I wished aunt Peggy was my mother because she let me do whatever I wanted to do. This caused turmoil between the sisters. It angered my mother to the point where she forbade me from spending so much time with my aunt. This was sort of hard to police because my room was right beside Aunt Peggy's. She had to pass through my room to access any part of the rest of the house and even to leave. Aunt Peggy moved out not long after this. I don't think I ever saw my aunt alive again; she was killed a few years later by a jealous boyfriend. Aunt Peggy just like mom was 5'2 or so and around 110 lbs., pretty almond complexion, and fiery. The story told to us was she was hell-bent on leaving the apartment one night to go partying with a girlfriend. He forbade her and threatened to kill her if she left. Before she could open the door he called her out of her name, and as she looked back to say that was the last bitch she'd be for him; he shot her with a 12 gauge shotgun in her abdomen, then sat and watched her writhe in pain for hours until the life drained from her small body. I'm not even sure if he ever served any time for that senseless killing. I do know that it affected my mother's sleep for months because she had to identify her younger sister's lifeless body at the Raleigh North Carolina morgue. At the funeral my mother broke down in a way that I've never seen before or ever again. I can only assume that she had many different emotions going on standing there knowing that she would never be able to go shopping for matching outfits or ride to work together ever again. No more long periods of silence on the phone just to never say those long overdue words: I miss you, I love you and most of all I'm sorry or please come home. Also, never seeing her killer brought to justice angered that feisty little woman to no end. It took all my father's knowledge and love to convince her not to take the law and revenge into her own hands. Luckily poetic justice prevailed before mom caught up with the man that killed my aunt. He died in an accident in his apartment three months after killing Aunt Peggy. The word was that trying to exit the bathtub after a shower he slipped and fell breaking his neck and wasn't found for many days until his rotting corpse finally drew attention. He succumbed to a heart attack. I can only hope that he suffered just as he forced my aunt to do.

I started school in the fall of 1971, at that time I still weighed 32 pounds at five years old. My overprotective mother used to follow the school bus every morning to every stop on Mrs. Brown's route. When Mrs. Brown realized what my mother was doing, she reported it to the school bus authorities and my mother was given an ultimatum: either trust her daughter to Mrs. Brown or become a school bus driver and transport me herself. This is exactly what she did, by the time summer school started she had gotten her school bus license. From June 1972 until her retirement in June 1991, my mother drove bus 18 and said this was the second most fulfilling job she had ever done. Second only to motherhood. I attended kindergarten at what became the administration building before moving onto Emporia Elementary school in fall of 72 where I met young Miss Prince. I don't know if I ever knew her first name because we only saw each other for 10 to 15 minutes in the afternoons while waiting to be dismissed on our buses. Little Miss Prince was a true princess to me because she looked just like a doll that I had received for Christmas even down to the silver tiara she wore to school every day. This particular day was the evening of picture day we both had on pretty white dresses and Patent-leather shoes (you know the ones with slick soles) we were chasing each other around the desks when she stumbled and fell hitting her head on the corner of a desk. I had never seen so much blood, they took her away in an ambulance and later that night I had nightmares. It happened on a Friday so on Saturday afternoon my mom contacted her mom to find out a few things; first to measure the atmosphere, to see if the whole family was as friendly and accepting as Little Miss Prince and to see if I could visit. I don't know if she cared so much about the girl's injuries (I know she did) but her main concern was my mentality. Another sleepless night and anxiety attack wasn't happening on her watch. Mom knew that I would not be okay until I saw that the girl was alive and going to live.

Another time fear crept into my mind was after Aunt Peggy's funeral. As I walked past some intimate garments on the inside clothesline, the things hanging there began to sway as if someone had walked past before me. I screamed for mom and asked if Aunt Peggy was there? I'm not sure if I'm afraid of ghosts but just as I thought it could have been Auntie or maybe that man that killed her because mom made it known that she was going to do what the judicial system failed to do; execute him just as he did my favorite auntie. Also there was a recurring dream about someone having a motorcycle accident near a drainage opening under a sidewalk. Somehow I was convinced that they crashed in such fashion that they spill across a busy street and slide down into the drainage opening. I don't know who or why but it became so polarizing that I was afraid to allow my feet to go near or under the side of my bed. It was so traumatizing that I would do everything in the middle of the floor, even kneeling on a stool by my dresser to say my prayers. After finishing my nightly routine I would dive from mid room into bed. Once I believe I knocked myself out because I hit my head on the wall when I misjudged my leap and can't remember anything from that point about that night.

I believe that its summer break before changing schools, because I'm wearing some navy blue shorts. I remember I received this bicycle for

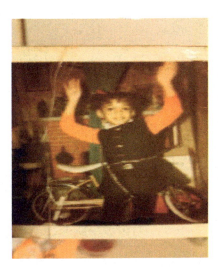

Christmas that year. I'm sure of this: had my parents known fostering my love of all things wheeled would've lead to so many accidents, I would have had to buy my own tricycle... LOL!!!

PAGE 20

Which I'm sure I probably took a few spills on that may have made this list if I could remember them. Back to this one, it's a weekend because dad is home. Probably another Saturday evening because he's got sawdust on his boots, I saw it when he scooped me up and rushed me indoors yelling for mommy. Forgive me, I've just jumped to the end, let's take a step or two back. Just as I've done thousands of times before I'm making circles around the house, from the side yard, down the side path, taking the long way around and back up the back path to the back yard. It's got to be my fourth trip. My mom's favorite outside dog is alongside me barking at the clickers on my front tire, suddenly he changed sides. Putting him on the inside between me and the corner of the house, so riding a little bit wider circle I ran into a stone sticking up out of the ground at just the precise angle to cause me to come to a dead stop, flip over the handlebars, fly awkwardly into the air and fall hard onto the handlebars which managed to perforate my hymen. Denying any possible lover the ultimate pleasure. I was bleeding profusely and crying like a naked newborn that just had their bottom smacked. This was also the start of my menstrual cycles. My mother rushed me to the emergency room to be told nothing was broken, other than pain medicine and iron supplements it would have to run its course. WOW! What a course it turned out to be I bled for two weeks straight, went off for exactly four days and started again. I think I lived in the doctor's office much more than most children because of ear aches, sore throats and colds. Although when doctors wanted to take out my tonsils my mom wouldn't sign the papers because she believed it would lead to needing further surgeries like tubes in my ears. My mom feared surgery for me or anyone especially because she went through breast cancer surgery in the summer of 1974 and hid it from everyone or maybe just me. I figured out something was going on when dad came to get me from grandma's house and stopped along the way to redo my hair; breaking down in tears when he couldn't figure out how to braid plats. He showed his vulnerability and expressed his fearful thoughts of being useless against something he had no control over. I didn't know how to help either one of them deal with this. Thankfully all turned out okay I assume because I never heard either one ever speak of that week ever again.

It's a cold day in November 1975, my daddy trusted me with the task of starting all of the cars that morning. I'm not sure what it is with the number three, but it seems that every accident happens about every three years. I don't remember being anything but excited. Everything went fine with the Pontiac, just simply turned the key. Wonderful now on to the baby of the bunch, the Plymouth, easy didn't even have to get totally in the driver's seat, easy turn of the key. Now on to the senior member of the fleet, the Caprice this car is almost twice my age and my daddy's favorite. He often referred to it as "Big Red" a lovable play on mom's nickname "Little Red". This Caprice was my dad's work in progress, not only has he rebuilt the engine to factory specs, he has already restored the interior to pristine showroom luster and now he's in the midst of redoing the exterior. One might ask, why? Why did my father trust me with his pride and joy? Or maybe even the biggest question of all, what happened? Well I'm not exactly sure, but here's to the best of my recollection what I did. I know that I had my backpack sitting on the top of the wood shed and I grabbed it as I skipped pass. Yes, skipping because my ego had swollen by now, feeling good because the other cars had started so easily, I'm sure I was thinking "this is too easy". Also knowing that mom was going to drive that car today and that we were leaving as soon as the car had heated up. This is where my problem ensued. I put the key into the ignition switch and turned expecting the same results, but to my dismay the only thing that came on was the radio and the windshield wipers. So I tried again. Reaching to turn down the radio, because I'm determined to do this myself. Remembering, that mom would pat the gas pedal three times and then retry, so I attempted to do this same thing. Having to scoot forward, I'm sure that I pulled myself forward by wrapping my arms around the steering wheel, which probably means I also gripped the gearshift as well. Thus placing the car in reverse. Now trying to start the car, sent the car rolling. Luckily my foot wasn't still on the gas, because it would have backed straight into my dad's logging truck. Oh yeah, you thought that was the accident didn't you? When I attempted to cover up having moved at all, I put the car in drive to pull forward a tiny bit, that's when I crashed into the fence, tangling a three foot tall metal fence in the undercarriage. You see children understand literal phrases; my daddy was the sweetest, most calm, fun loving soul you could ever meet. But he took his vehicles as seriously as protecting his family. He considered them a part of the family I'm almost certain, especially "Big Red". Around town many people didn't know him by name but if you said the man with the clean red trucks they would know who you were talking about immediately. Not that I thought dad would do anything to me about damaging his precious work in progress, I'm a parent pleaser or even people in general. So much so that I've always put others feelings before mine. Instead of going and saying I had a problem cranking "Big Red" I tried to get it free myself. I'm not sure if I was trying to be independent, or if it's just ashamed. Nonetheless, to add injury to insult (yes I'm aware I've reversed the typical order) in attempting I cut my hand really deep requiring stitches and a tetanus shot.

Every report card that I got over the years said the same thing in the comment section, Kimberly is a bright student, but could use her time more wisely and could spend less time talking. This occupied the comment section from kindergarten through the fourth grade. My teacher even failed me one half grade in the fourth, so where I should have been going to the fifth I had to repeat half of the fourth grade again. Thankfully the teacher I had that year, Mr. Harrell, would have no part in partial completion. Mr. Harrell recognized the fact that I was just under challenged, so when I finished my regularly assigned task or homework, he would challenge me with work from a higher grade. So in the fall of 77 I started the sixth grade. There have been times that my mom threatened to come to school and paddle me in front of the class to teach me a lesson or to shame me into keeping my mouth shut. Little did anybody know most of my talking in class was to tell others to leave me alone during a test I didn't want to get anyone in trouble and I wasn't going to help anyone on their test? Not to brag on myself but I always found the lessons that the teachers were teaching to be very easy. I hardly ever had to study as long as I paid attention in class and did my homework. Unfortunately because of this I was bullied for many years. Girls used to hate me because I developed early and boys liked it. Boys were too touchy-feely and girls hated all of the attention the boys showed me. So I found myself alone in most situations. I believe because of all of the isolation I created my own world in books. I began to write poetry and love to create short stories. If only I had been able to hold on to all of the stuff that I wrote from third grade forward I might have enough for a nice book by now. As a matter of fact my writing was the cause of the first fight I ever had in school on Monday

April 1, 1974. I remember the date as if it was yesterday because:

1. It was April fool's day.
2. Tammy scared me by sneaking up behind.
3. She needed stitches and an ambulance.
4. This was my first appearance in the principal's office.

But most of all, my mother was notified, even though she was told I wasn't being expelled or even disciplined. You see Tammy was the class bully and got what she was asking for or maybe a little more. Tammy was the granddaughter of the most influential bigot of our town. Mr. Snodgrass owned the main Central Fidelity Bank, the Star Value grocery, and sat on the board of every healthcare facility in town. It was no mystery how he felt about black folks, you could hear him say often "Niggers can only shine my shoes before I step on them." Although many colored people had bank accounts with Central Fidelity banks it was an unwritten rule that in order to keep your money affairs safe you used any one of the other branches. If he could he would not allow pennies to be stored in the vault. His attitude infected his whole family's psyche, even the youth. Tammy was a chip off that old block. Bitch, coon and nigger flew out of her mouth faster than good morning. That day, every boy in class had some stupid trick to cop a sneaky feel or an all on groping. So none of us wanted to deal with Tammy's badgering and name calling. I warned her after the first statement she uttered that morning to go away but, NO! You see this revenge was sanctioned by Mrs. Brown before lunch. Teacher's couldn't reach out and touch students but they knew how to look the other way at the precise moments. On the way to the cafeteria Mrs. Brown chose me to head the line to and from the cafeteria; even after I had my turn the previous week. An honor or a set-up? To a 9 year old teacher's pet it was an honor and a curse; I knew someone wasn't going to be happy. At lunch I sat alone and after I did exactly what Mrs. Brown asked led the class back to the classroom. As usual the teacher went to the supply closet to retrieve art supplies. This created the perfect window for Tammy. She knocked everything off my desk, my books, pencils, calculator and my brand new glasses; everything flew in different directions. When I attempted to stand up from my desk Tammy stepped in front of me, I stumbled backwards knocking over my desk and nearly fell myself. There was an embarrassingly loud crash from the desk and explosive laughter from my other classmates. To add insult to injury, Tammy is now standing too close for comfort, spouting something that I'm too angry to stop and understand, before thinking I grabbed the desk and swung for the fences. I only hit her once but it was enough to cause a concussion and split the side of her temple from eye socket to ear. From that day on until 7th grade I never had any more problems. Unfortunately Tammy proved to be a slow learner and kept picking on others.

I was always an awkward gangly kid who loved sports. I was always most at home on the monkey bars on the playground during recess. When we got stuck inside because of bad weather, I always wanted to swing on the rings. Eventually our gym teacher figured out everyone's strengths so that his whole class could pass the Presidential Physical Endurance Test, he would break us up into groups of four, as long as we each did one activity, we all passed. My mother probably wished they had adopted a more girly girl but my dad loved my tomboy side; I grew up with all the sporting equipment ever made, one mention of a game and dad built the space. I noticed a basketball one Saturday in W. T. Tiller and came home with it and the backboard and hoop. We had a huge yard and just as soon as I expressed interest in baseball he created a baseball field and invested in enough equipment for a team; never mind the fact that I didn't have enough friends to fill one side. My parents both bent over backwards to keep me happy because they felt I was lonely. I wasn't sure what was missing, if anything. I just think because they were older thought I needed a sibling. They once became foster parents to two boys but that didn't last long. The boys were identical twins that had been just removed from an abusive mother, so they didn't trust anyone and stuck to each other like they were glued at the hip. They wouldn't eat or talk so rather than admit that she was in over her head—my mother sent the boys away. My parents were in the midst of adopting another girl Gloria. I know she came from the adoption agency that I was from. Again they worked with Maxine Carter to have their perfect family. A week into this placement Gloria and I were playing in front of the living room door and she fell out and down some cement steps. She didn't seem injured but on our way to grandma's that Saturday I got mad because Gloria stopped playing with me and I told mom. We pulled over and an ambulance took her and mom to the hospital. She had a severe concussion and passed away later that Sunday. Mom took it hard, but saw it as a sign that our family was as it should remain. I never heard another mention of expanding. She saw it as another blemish on her perfect record.

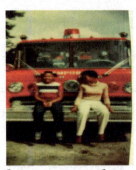

My parents were best friends with the Jarrell's and they had three children, two boys and a daughter. They figured this was the closest thing to siblings they'd be able to give me. We used to go places together on the weekends with the Jarrell's. The first weekend both sets of parents drove their own vehicles but by the following weekend my dad purchased a used black van. He worked on it every evening after work to get it road ready so that we all could ride together whenever we went anywhere on those weekend jaunts. I can't say every outing was fun but they'd were interesting. I didn't realize this one time when we stopped at the fire station was because one of the mom's had a medical issue going on; I still to this day don't know which one. Mama and Mrs. Jarrell had been friends before but became closer after Aunt Peggy moved out; thankfully so because mom was so sad after her death. I only remember that the fathers and we children went on our way to their favorite fishing hole for that week's outing. I only remember our dads being quiet all that day, not their usually joking big brother and little brother attitudes.

I don't understand why every boy is wired the same. The conversation on the fire truck was about sex and her brothers were no different. Every time we were together the older brother would try to pinch me somewhere inappropriate and pretend it was an accident. The younger brother hadn't quite figured out his hormones but knew he wanted to be wherever I was, this made him the fun, adventurous one. Whatever stupid thing I was getting into he was my sidekick. Always! I got into the craziest things like once getting my finger stuck in a bottle at a lake that had some of the grossest smelling pond scum in it that spilled all over my hand. It stunk to high heaven and no matter how much I washed my hands it seemed to intensify. No one else would sit near me for the rest of the trip but Patches didn't desert me.

King's Dominion opened in May of 1975 that was the year I begged to go to summer school. I learned that hanging out with mom everyday wasn't all it was cracked up to be. Riding the bus was meant only for to and from school for a reason, especially for a child with no control of the activities of the day and no concept of time. At least at school there's activities, school work, lunch and even tests; all better than trying to amuse myself for 6 hours a day without being able to do many different things. I missed my bicycle, dogs, outside time and different toys. My mom didn't like me interacting with the other children and I was afraid to join into conversations with the adults unless asked something. So I would sit in the back of the bus alone until asked to join. This too seemed wrong because the other drivers would be shocked to see me or would change their tone or the entire conversation. I didn't realize that my decision to attend summer school that year would open up a slot for my friend to go to Kings Dominion with us. I know things work the way God plans. It was great to have a girl's day. That next June we went back on one of our weekend outings with the whole Jarrell clan but it wasn't as fun for us girls because we had to do stuff that the boys wanted to do. I think that I started acting more girly after hanging out with Tessie. Maybe that was my mom's intent, but my dad saw his "Chap" slipping away. I felt the tug of war between them and didn't like it. I didn't want the disappointed look from either one of them. I think I learned the art of manipulation during that time.

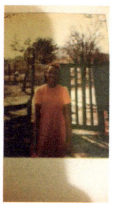
I know parents love living vicariously through their children. They enroll us in all the activities that are supposed to shape us into well-rounded adults. One of those things I was forced into was our church choir. As a matter of fact, I'm sure everything I understood about religious practices were because my parents dropped me at Sunday school every Sunday morning and choir practice every Wednesday night. My parents attended church on the second Sunday of every month because children's choir was the featured entertainment. I guess me being one of the go to soloists would not look so good without my mom's well timed happy holy ghost filled weep session during my rendition of Amazing Grace or her saying sing it baby during any other songs. I'm quite sure I continued to go to church because that's what had been required of me. I even got baptized at the age 11 on March 19, 1978, the week before Easter. I was told this was the perfect age to receive the blessing of the Lord. Now looking back I'm realizing this is the only place my parents felt

comfortable enough sending me without being with me or maybe this was the only alone time they could steal.

I also used to love playing volleyball and I had a wicked serve that no one could return. Back when I was in junior high or high school we didn't have a volleyball team in my school. We only had the football and basketball teams for the boys. I wasn't into basketball but I joined the track team in junior high which was the only sports related thing girls could participate in. During the eighth grade staying after school one day for track practice, catching the late activity bus was when I spotted the man that I thought I would spend the rest of my life with. He was handsome, mysterious, and smelled so good. Even though it was the end of the day, he looked as though he had gotten dressed just to meet me. I on the other hand was winded, sweaty and tired from track practice when I got on the bus, it was all I could do to collapse in the seat. We made eye contact as I sat down and I could feel the tingle of a blush as I smiled. Until now I had not even given guys a second look, but this was no ordinary guy.

For a whole summer I went on with my normal activities not even giving him another thought. That summer I had band practice every day. From 9 AM until 3 PM every day we marched back and forth in the hot sun, trying to get ready for the first football game of the year. Our first game was always at home so the band performed during the halftime show. And the second Saturday in September was always the Peanut Festival Parade. I always got stuck in the positions I hated either carrying the American flag during the football games or carrying the school banner during parades. Although both positions were easy and important they always seemed to come at the wrong time. I wouldn't be prepared for the role that I got drafted for at the last minute. I became the flag carrier on the night of the first dance when I was expecting to be just another rifleman so I showed up dressed in my performance skirt to be told to go search the uniform closet for some pants because the flagman had to be in full uniform, it was still 74° outside that night and steaming hot in the gym during the dance (to which I was stuck in full uniform) I wanted to attend. Another time I showed up really ready to embrace the flagman's role because we were doing the Christmas parade in Roanoke Rapids North Carolina and it was 34° when we boarded the bus. Thankfully my mom believed in being prepared but nothing could prepare me for the cruelest section leader and the harshness of the weather that day. I had suspicions that more than bad luck was behind my "short straw luck" of the time. That time Cecilia just knew she had won, she waited until we'd left the school to tell me I'd be carrying the banner in the parade knowing this meant I was overdressed because our banner girls wore the shortest skirts. I asked why she waited until that moment to tell me. Only because I wanted to see if she had the courage to admit bullying me because she was mad that the guy she drooled over chose to sit next to me during a long bus ride to Carey N.C. over the summer. Little did she know I was no more interested in (C.M) than He was in girls! I exited the bus and made my way to the bathroom emerging looking like I came knowingly and willingly ready for that crazy girl's bullshit. As I walked pass I heard her best friend laugh at her and say "damn girl she got your man and your number"—I felt vindicated as everyone in her little click laughed. If I could have I probably would have ran screaming back to the warmth of daddy's truck because by the time we got to our destination the cold drizzle had turned to ice crystals – it was coming down pants and long johns kind of weather. I took solace in the fact that

Cecilia was just as cold as I was. Maybe her anger was enough to warm her—just as seeing her humiliated, warmed me. The slight drizzle has turned into ice coming down harder than snow. Even though I was wearing two pair of stockings and thick white gloves I'd rather be still in long pants

Chapter 2: **The Change**

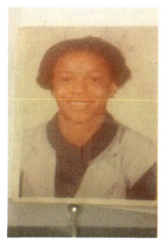

In 1979 I became a big girl and a woman all in the same month. My freshman year at Greensville County high school I was a member of the hall patrol. I think I liked this appointment because I got to leave class early, arrive at my next class late, boss people around, and write people up. It was during one of my patrolmen assignments that I spotted "Mr. Right" again, as a matter of fact I threatened to write him up for hanging out in the halls after the bell has sounded. This was my lame attempt at flirting, but it worked. When arriving at my fourth period class a classmate and my table mate was standing in the doorway talking to my mystery man. I soon found out that he was her brother it was on and cracking. I know that she got tired of me asking questions about her brother, but I had to know anything that she would share. Betty introduced us and it was the beginning of a beautiful a little love affair. When Willie and I first started dating he was 15 and would ride his bicycle the 7 miles to my house. We would stay on the phone and talk for hours when we were not together. We would have the most profound conversations about anything and everything, it was as a budding relationship should be. We spent time learning about each other. He learned that I was spoiled and loved to be spoiled and I learned that he was insanely jealous, nonetheless I still loved spending time with him. I know that he also helped to foster my love of writing. Mom and dad took us everywhere they went exposing us to grown folk life. My mother was an Eastern star and their annual Christmas pageant was held in Virginia Beach. This was the first time I was ever allowed to have a mixed drink with dinner. We ate, we drank, and we danced the night away. On the ride home in the back of the van I laid with my head in Willie's lap, my head spinning a little from the E and J and Coke. I could smell his overpowering essence through his pristine creased blue pinstriped pants, I became bolder than ever. I

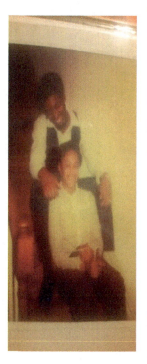 just had to taste him, so I gave him one of the best BJ's he had ever had. I'm not sure if my parents knew what was going on just behind the driver's seat. I can only think that they did not because neither one of them said anything when we got home or maybe they were just so horrified that they just didn't know what to say. Looking back now, and knowing the kind of person my mother was this is not something that I am proud of. Young love will make you do a lot of things you may look back on and wonder why? I have often asked myself did I do the things that I did hoping not to lose him to someone else or what? Sometimes you can live your life too fast, when you take time to slow down. When you look back you just want to go back and tell your young self you're crazy. Another time when my parents decide to visit my Uncle Snake for Easter break, they allowed Willie to go along, this is the trip we took the staircase picture. Willie and I were in my uncle's basement drinking shots of "Cutty Sark" and where there was alcohol there was sex. We were so in love then, young, dumb, and full of fun.

Sometimes we do things without thinking about the consequences, living in the moment, satisfying the flesh. Obeying those unwritten rules were not even on our minds. Not necessarily trying to live on a wild side, at that young age I know I just loved him. My mom realized that her little girl was changing into a demonstrative young lady that she could no longer control.

One evening when we set out going to the movies, Willie and I, Betty and her boyfriend, we only made it 3mi. from their house before … In my defense, I was trying to prevent a head on collision. Also, I wasn't driving, I was busy looking for a new package of rolling papers. Yeah I'm aware it's not sounding so good yet. *Well please hold all condemnation until the close of this summation.* Together during this situation was my boyfriend of a year and a half, his sister and her boyfriend in the backseat. The conversation was about the wrestling match that we had attended the previous weekend. Instead of passing the weed back to Carl, my man just knew he could do it all; teach me how to remove the seeds, roll a decent joint, and drive at the same time. Well of course Little Miss Naïve Me, wasn't doing it properly (might I add didn't care), so I exclaimed "do it yourself then" and passed everything over. In bringing my arm back, I hit the book of paper which slid between my seat and the center console. I bent down to retrieve the fallen papers and sat up just in time to see us drifting into the path of a dump truck. So I grabbed the steering wheel and jerked. Startling everyone as we felt the breeze of the zooming truck, unaware that I'd over corrected ran onto the soft shoulder of the right side of the road and into the ditch. It was such a quick right to left jerking that the weed spilled and the tire blew. Forcing the car to spin and by this time my hand was off of the wheel. I could not understand why no one else reacted to the approaching truck, maybe the music was too loud to hear the horn. As I'm reviewing the facts, maybe this should not even be called an accident. Yes, it caused damages to the car but we all walked away unhurt. "Any accident you walked away from is just an incident" so my dad used to say. Let my boyfriend tell it, I may have saved us but I'm on the hook for hurting his precious "first baby". After I reminded him that he should have been paying attention to the road instead of weed, he got over himself.

It is early April 1982, one Saturday morning, mom is in the kitchen cooking breakfast and I walk into the kitchen and immediately get sick from the smell of eggs cooking. I run to the bathroom and start to throw up. Immediately my mom follows me and gives me this look of discontent and says "you're pregnant." She then returns to the kitchen and finishes cooking breakfast, slamming pans and pots. She makes a phone call and tells me "we're going to see the doctor." A few hours later it was officially confirmed I was three weeks pregnant. After the silent treatment the rest of the day, Sunday morning shortly after breakfast I was given three options: First Option go to my uncle's house in Maryland and have an abortion and then come home or second option go to my Uncle's and have the baby and put it up for adoption or third option get the hell out of her house. Well, given my own situation having been adopted myself I didn't want to subject my own child to that and I did not believe in abortions, so my only option was to leave. Fearing the result of telling school authorities that my mom put me out of the house because of the pregnancy, I made up a story that my father had been molesting me since age eight. I know now how bad this story could have been but at the time I didn't know what else to do. All day that Monday I was crying during classes and Vice Principal Mrs. Young saw me at my locker and brought me to her office and asked me what was wrong. This is when that made up story came spilling out. Right about now is when it dawns on me that my big girl life just became an adult one. I went from being a 15-year-old girl to being a pregnant homeless adult.

For five months I've bounced around from foster home to foster home. It is now September the beginning of a new school year, I am as big as the house, and I feel out of place and alone. Even though things seem to be settling down I've been in this foster home for almost a month now and as she is known affectionately as Aunt Mary by the other foster children. She has told me that even though she wishes it could be a permanent placement but this is yet another temporary one. Unfortunately one bad apple can spoil the whole bunch. There is one foster child here that causes problems for all of us and in order to get rid of him she has to get rid of all of us. So in the meantime I will just make do. This is the first foster placement that I have shared a room it's a huge upstairs bedroom with two full size beds, two writing desks, and an oil heater. Being the spoiled person that I am, although Phyllis is a decent person, I do not like sharing a room. I found out today that I am due in December, Dr. Healy is predicting Christmas. On my way home from the doctor's office I walked past Deanne's consignment shop, just as I have every two weeks prior but today I can finally purchase that pretty pink layette set they have in the window because Dr. Healy said I'm having a girl. Finally, someone to love me the way that I will love them.

It was December 9th and last night the baby kept waking me from any type of restful positions. I've heard people say "I was just pulling your leg" referring to a funny story, but the baby took it literally. Every time I would fall deep asleep, I'd be jerked awake by leg twitches. Looking back now, I realize that God was sparing me the humiliation of my water breaking before even reaching school that morning. You see because I was dog tired and famished when it was time to get ready for school. I decided to take that day to ready the room, clean from top to bottom, and assemble the crib. First things first: A lumberjack breakfast which included scrambled eggs, bacon, toast, and OJ. Breakfast was great, I cleaned kitchen, then went back upstairs for the task at hand. No sooner than I placed both feet on the carpeting at the top of the long staircase, the telephone rings. Feeling no pain, actually feeling quite satisfied from breakfast, I answered the telephone laughing. Laughter quickly turned into concern because as I greeted the caller my water broke. My mom was on the other end grilling me about why wasn't I at school. It's barely past the first bell. Mom had to have been informed by C. Richards that I wasn't on the bus that morning. Even out of her house my mother had spies that kept her abreast of my every move. This time I wasn't mad at her. I ran to the downstairs bathroom where I met with opposition, Jewel the one housemate that rented from Aunt Mary. Usually I put up with her quirky attitude but this morning her refusal to yield the bathroom cut through me roughly, before even thinking I ripped her a line unworthy of repeating. The mama bear in me growled as if someone just threatened bodily harm to my soon to be born cub. I can only assume nerves have taken over my normally peaceful demeanor, because until now being pregnant only meant I couldn't wear tight jeans, now being a mother is becoming real and is no longer a novel abstract idea. Sensing the urgency of the fact that my water broke an hour ago I need to make my way to the hospital. Unfortunately there is no one in the house and I have to walk to the nearest neighbor's house which is a half football field away. Aunt Irene is Aunt Mary's sister she lives next door and luckily she works the night shift and is at home preparing to go to sleep. The two sister's work as nurses at Greensville Memorial Hospital the very hospital I am headed to.

I have been laying here since 9:45 this morning and nothing else has happened. Dr. Healy came to visit and to check my progress after doing an exam he told me he was going to play nine holes of golf, maybe by that time I will have dilated enough to start pushing. Right about now all I want to do is walk down the hall to my first period class which is held here at the hospital. I need to notify Ms. Owens that I'm in here as a patient. We had hoped that I wouldn't go into labor until the Christmas break so that I wouldn't miss any school because before the break we would have her mid-semester exam. My grades are decent but no grade can withstand a zero on an exam. The nurses come in every hour on the hour to chart my progress and prep me for the actual blessed event. At lunch time I was allowed to eat lunch but as soon as I was finished the nurse came in to give me an enema, start an IV, and inform me that I was NPO (nothing by mouth) from this point on because I have dilated to 5 cm and it should be any time now. Luckily Ms. Owens knew that I was always in class and the only time I would miss class would be to give birth, so when I didn't show up for class she checked the inpatient list and came to see me after everyone had gone on break. That day just happened to be one of our training days and instead of having a patient load I became one of my classmate's patients to care for. Because my water had broken, not only was I NPO I could not get out of bed, so every time I had to go to the bathroom I had to call the nurse for the bed pan. At 2 o'clock "General Hospital" came on TV and Laura was giving birth to her son and I looked at it and said "why is she pretending that this is so hard, she pretended that she was in such pain, what a wonderful actress." You see I still haven't had any quote "labor pains" yet. Even when the monitor shows that I'm having a labor wave it has not hurt. Little did I know what I was in for, because by 4 o'clock I was deep in the throes of labor pains I don't know if they coincided with the fact that my mother had gotten there and was playing helicopter mom. Each time I had a labor pain my mom wanted me to hold her hand I kept saying no but this one time before I could grip the rail she had gripped my hand. You see I don't think she thought about this very well because she wore rings on every finger and some fingers two or three rings. To put her hand in mine meant sheer and utter pain for the both of us for about five minutes. Unfortunately, I was told by the nurse that I couldn't have anything for pain until I was dilated to 8 cm for some reason this took until 11:45 PM. Eight hours of sheer terror, crying because I wanted water, was in pain, and was being annoyed by my mother. All I wanted other than relief was to see Willie. When they finally gave me pain medicine at midnight I cried myself to sleep thinking that he didn't care enough to show up. My mother knew I wanted to see him but she never told me he was there or went to get him. Why didn't she tell me he was there? Another chance for her to control the situation. To assert her dominance. To prove she was still in control of my life.

When I woke up it was 4:55 AM- I was in excruciating pain again, the nurse checked me and told me it was time. I was then taken into the labor and delivery room, still never knowing that

Willie was even in the hospital. I had to go through this with nobody but the doctors, nurses and my mother. Back then I wasn't as strong as I am now; if I had it to do over again I would've made a stink, I would've raised my voice, I would've made sure that Willie was in that room. I think that there were a few times in our relationship that could've been pivotal moments in time, I think that was one. Just like a lot of others I kept quiet and missed opportunities to change my future one way or the other. My beautiful baby boy yes, I said baby boy was born at 5:55 AM on Friday December 10, 1982. Needless to say, I wasn't prepared for that one. You see, the only thing I brought to the hospital to take my baby home in was that pretty pink layette set that one from the consignment shop five months ago. After making sure that he had all 10 fingers and all 10 toes I think I went back to sleep for a few hours, needless to say I was wiped out. Every day the nurses worked with me to make sure that I knew how to take care of the baby. They taught me how to hold him, care for his umbilicus, prepare formula, and change diapers. Back in the day they didn't toss you out on your head as soon as you had the baby they actually made sure that you were doing okay. My postpartum care was interesting because I had stitches in the front and in the back. Even though Pete only weighed 7 lbs. 15 oz. I was split from coast-to-coast. So moving around is going very slow. We were in the hospital a full week after he was born until Saturday, December 18th. My mother had to go to a gift shop to buy a boys outfit for him to be able to take pictures and have some clothes on his back when we went home. Pete must have known it was going to be hard for us because he was a good baby hardly ever cried. The only time was when he was hot. Like a typical mother I would over dress him, in my defense it was December and at some point while we were in the hospital it snowed really bad. Also, like an overwhelmed mother it took me a while to figure out why he was crying. It wasn't until he started sweating that I figured out that he didn't like heat. Of course everyone assumed I was refusing or too lazy to dress my son, not at all, I like peace and quiet and a cool baby was a happy baby. Once Pete was hospitalized with Bronchitis when he was 4 months old, because he was exposed to a marijuana smoke filled room while the babysitter partied. This taught me that I couldn't go anywhere I couldn't take a baby. I've always been a trusting sort, but I became paranoid "ironic right" about leaving my precious child with anybody under the age of 30 after that.

One day after returning to school from spring break, I spotted my mother sitting in the ICU waiting room, she was slumped over using her coat and purse as a pillow in her lap. She informed me that my father had been admitted on Sunday night. That Sunday they'd tried to carry on a family tradition by going driving no particular place. After 2 hours and an ice cream cone later, they turned back into the driveway. As he always did going slowly because our dogs would run beside the vehicles, you would have to straddle the right edge of the driveway all the way up because of the neighbor's fence on the left. Once in his usual parking spot, mom said she went inside expecting my father to be behind her shortly. After preparing lunch for the next day which took about 30 minutes she realized that she's still hearing the sound of the van motor running. So she poked her head out and screamed "are you alright." Never getting an answer she went to check on him. Having to walk all the way around to the passenger's side to gain entrance concerned her. My father was in the midst of a stroke. She had no choice but to wrestle him into the passenger seat alone and drive him the 30 miles to the hospital in Emporia because to wait for emergency transportation would take more precious time than she could risk. Country living can be peaceful in good times but detrimental during a crisis. I can't ever remember seeing my mother looking so helpless ever before or after. I also remember feeling responsible for him being there. Had my lies caused his stroke? I didn't know how to comfort mom, or even how to be around her then. I tried to just distance myself from the truth that I was feeling because if I was feeling this way I knew mom was blaming me too. I went into his intensive care room and I can't remember what was on my mind exactly but I knew I didn't like being at his bedside seeing all the tubes, the two IV pumps and the respirator. I knew that wasn't how I wanted to see him or remember him. I barely mustered up, I'm sorry and ran out. I didn't want to face anyone from the family so I didn't even go to his funeral three weeks later. So ashamed and hurting I waited until mom made the first move to reach out for any kind of relationship.

Reality, depression, loneliness and isolation became my closest friends these past few weeks.

Everyone my age was thinking about prom, graduation or college prep classes over the summer. My first and foremost thought was that I wanted this next move to be my very last. Woke up to the news that the room I was renting was not going to be available anymore after May's end. Apparently not washing dinner dishes into the wee hours behind grown folk and forgetting to empty the diaper pail twice in two weeks, makes you trifling, filthy, and unworthy of a $50 a month room. So yet again 16 and homeless. At this time I'm an emancipated minor "oops" guess I fell asleep in class when that lesson was taught. I don't know which is harder to forgive and forget being uninformed or knowingly allowing havoc to occur.I have been wrestling with this for 34 years. I so wanted to be the best mom I could, for six months and two more foster homes I struggled with postpartum depression myself. Unfortunately, I had no idea what it was. Between classes, a sick child, getting sick myself and being misdiagnosed repeatedly, the depression went unattended for years. Sometimes I think that I never got over that bout of depression. Even right today, sometimes I can have crying episodes attached to feelings from my first pregnancy, which is strange because I've had three pregnancies since and two other children as a result. Maybe what I'm suffering from is separation anxiety. Although my son was not put up for adoption we were split apart when he was six months old. Luckily I had a great relationship with his grandmother on his father's side. This wasn't what I'd hoped for but being a single mom at 16 isn't easy... It's hard to feel that you fell short of expectations of all that you wish loved you unconditionally. Having a child of your own is a great responsibility. Now I find myself in the same position that my birth mother was in. One can appreciate and understand what she went through when faced with the same scenario.

I've accepted that things happened according to GOD's grand design. One can't help wonder what if? Had I fully understood emancipation maybe just maybe? I didn't know back then that since my father had been in the military that I was entitled to his social security benefits and my social worker chose to withhold this information also. I might have been able to survive in Emporia but oh well no need dwell on past events now.

Now the harshness of winter is budging reluctantly giving way to more gentle breezes, flowering trees, and pollen of spring. Sneezing or not, at least I can put the baby in the stroller and go. I gathered what we'd need to stay away all day. I walked all the way to Mitchell Brothers, then to A&P, then onto VEC in search of three things:

1. Affordable housing that allowed babies.
2. A babysitter
3. A job to pay for 1 & 2.

At sixteen I never thought about combining all and becoming a nanny. I've been babysitting for Miss April and her husband for two months and I hate it. Naw! This was too much like being a maid. My hats off to every Nanny, babysitter, maid, girl-Friday, ma'am or any other name someone who cares for other's houses and children are referred.

Don't get me wrong, I love children in a controlled environment like a daycare where I can care for them, cuddle them, and kick them out until next time. So much for that rant, Please forgive the stumbles over feelings that will happen from time to time in the telling of a true story. I'm running out of time and having no results alone, I ask my social worker for help in finding a place that would take me and the baby together. I'm hoping for an unwed mothers group home. Something got lost in translation. "Oh hell NO" nothing got lost except ME. I was told: "The shelter I wanted to go to didn't have a slot for me just yet because I have already delivered." Having been pressured into leaving Pete with his grandmother for a temporary placement until this imaginary placement opened up, my mother perpetrated her ultimate betrayal that day. I was out of her one horse town without my son. Now, not only alone, but I was in an institution for hardcore detainees, South Boston Detention Center. Supposedly I'm here for less than a week and then on to the placement requested and reunited with my baby. Another lie. June 3, 1983 its dusk and I was summoned to the transfer room. On to whatever else Barbara Walker had decided I should endure for her to feel vindicated, bad part about it my social worker had two faces but no spine. Why such secrecy, just as suspected not somewhere my baby can come to live. This time I'm told you're here until 18+ (possible for 2 year program). It's now 9:15PM just enough time to make my bed with this issued set given, hear all the household rules, go to the bathroom and go to bed at 10. After looking back, I realized my birthday was on Sunday, which meant family visits. Another feather in "dear old Mumsie's" hat because I had set up a visit with Willie, his parents, and my bundle of Joy. My mother was a real piece of work when angered. This being said, aren't we all. I'm probably falling short in the eyes of GOD right now with this paragraph. Oh well, if I've learnt nothing else this year, I definitely learned to try my best at using the system to my advantage. New surroundings, new set of rules, but at least it doesn't feel like mom is controlling the people in charge. This is a group home yes, but not a detention center. The girls home is part of a collective set called "the Community Attention Groups." There's another house a few blocks away that holds up to 25 boys at any given time. This three story old Victorian has seven bedrooms, two recreation rooms one equipped with a pool table, a huge twenty seat eat-in kitchen, the living room also has seating for fifteen but surface area to retrieve chairs from other rooms and still not feel crowded. Like most houses there never seem to be enough closet space or bathrooms. Each of the bedrooms on the main and upstairs floors held at least two beds. I hated the shared room experience because privacy and individuality got lost. The basement bedrooms were singles that for the most part was unmonitored by staff. After finding this out I've

> GOD forgive my attitude. I'm working hard to change, to forgive, to let go and let YOU work it out! But I'm human... We

got one mission in mind, earning my levels quickly.

Each "newbie" started out the same with no privileges for the first two weeks on level 1, you could go out with staff or an upper level resident but your curfew was 8:30PM. Earning your next level wasn't hard but holding on to it was sometimes challenging. Keeping your levels depended on your willingness to grow as a young lady, productive member of the program and society. So shutting down into your own pitiful life wasn't allowed. You had to do your assigned chores for a week straight which was easier than talking or writing in my journal every day. Quite often I found myself writing about home and how alone I felt quite often. (If I'd been able to hold on to those journals I'd be further along with this book now.) A plan of action was required on/in Wednesday's journal entry. Going home for the weekend was my plan every week, but mostly only happened one weekend a month. You always had to continuously work toward achieving your ultimate goals. My goal was always to reconnect my family. Me, my baby and his father. Little did I know, that GOD's plan would take me in such different directions, I often wonder about nature verses nurture and whether my naturally flirty demeanor was the deciding factor. I didn't lose sight of my goals they just started to look unattainable. Separation does nothing for love; sometimes you cannot see the forest for the trees. Traveling home every weekend was out of the realm of possibility but I tried to make it home every two weeks, but I wasn't strong enough to assert my feelings and wishes so I lost the love of my life to someone that pretended to be my best friend. It became increasingly harder to come home on Friday evenings knowing as soon as I stepped off the Greyhound at 9:05PM the clock started my countdown until Sunday at 2PM when the return trip ascended upon any happiness I could be having. On Friday's we received our allowance of $5, if you had fulfilled your weekly goals. The weekends were pretty laidback, most of the times we had these "pushover" relief staffers that we could talk into an outing, such as a movie, swimming, or the mall that had an arcade for a few hours of freedom from the same old routine of playing pool for hours. On most weekends that I got stuck in the city I voluntarily worked on my off weekends at Eldercare Gardens.

Sometimes on these long bus rides you can meet the most interesting people but mostly I was wishing for more time. I did make friends with an Army serviceman that always seemed to be traveling every time I was. I often wonder whatever happened to Robin D. Dixon. This was during the Reagan days, hopefully he didn't get sent overseas to fight in that senseless war. Maybe after I find my family the next search will be for Robin. He would always be on the bus when I boarded in Richmond headed to his mother's in North Carolina. I realized talking to Robin made the time go by easier going and he was the one that soothed the tears away on the return trip. I remember looking at him fondly after one conversation thinking **wow** there's actually another guy that makes me feel something out here. Also I realized something that my ex had accused me of was looking more like the truth… just not as bad as he claimed. He believed I was prejudiced against light skinned brothers. I only think we all have our preferences, maybe some should be more in touch with what our wants and needs are. Robin was average height but under 6' ft. I always saw him in his dress uniform and polished dress shoes. He always had this intoxicating manly smell, infectious smile and tantalizing conversation. Damn now that I think back I can remember the sadness I felt when he and I traveled on the opposite weekends. We exchanged information, corresponded some but I didn't write as much as he did. Maybe subconsciously I still held a torch for my ex and didn't foster what could've been with Robin. I still have the pictures he sent in the family album. We drifted apart when I got sick and didn't return to Charlottesville immediately after Easter and no one gave me his last letter until three months later. I would pray for Robin every night and drift off smiling.

Chapter 3: The ongoing health issues

When I went home for Easter break in 1984, still having stomach problems that hadn't been properly diagnosed I became deathly ill. I was riding with my mom on her elementary school run but I got off just in time to throw up. I looked like Linda Blair without my head turning 360°. The emesis was dark green and I filled a quart jar and a bath basin to the top within ten minutes, by the time I finished. I was rushed to the hospital, just to hangout another week under observation and undergoing tests. I remember being so sick that I was on a clear liquid diet and not even being able to keep it down. Of course I needed pain medicine every six hours and doctors had no problem with that, it was me with the issues. There was only two options, injection longer acting, stronger, and recommended or pills: less effective, don't last as long, and barely took the edge off. Well, being as terrified of needles as I am, I endured the pain as long as I could before asking for anything for relief. I got the injection only once, although it worked very well and I was finally able to fall off to sleep for a good amount of time. The next time I could get medicine for pain I opted for the pills. Finally after being tethered to my bed for 5 days by extreme pain and an IV in the top of my left hand, they figured out what had been bothering me for almost 2 years now. Everyone that I have saw about my condition chalked it up to stress. Finally, a diagnosis, and immediately surgery to remove my gall bladder. Doctor Sedki a tenacious Asian American doctor that migrated to Emporia some twenty years prior was the go to expert on mysterious medical conditions said "You are my youngest client to ever need this surgery, but I'll fix you right up." I was 17 years old and had seventeen stones. They ranged in size from a small pearl to a Brazil nut. Doctor Sedki put them into a large specimen cup for me to be able to keep, but mom purposely left them behind the day I went home. After surgery I couldn't even move by myself for a few days. Back then surgeons didn't worry so much about what the scar left behind would look like, just as long as they got you well. I proudly sport a foot long scar across my abdomen because my incision got ripped open a week and 3 days after I had surgery. Vanity gave way to a scared son. I had been told not to lift anything weighing more than 5lbs. for as long as my incision was healing. Pete and I were outside in the front yard playing with a basketball unaware that Shanghai his father's six month old Doberman Pincher was not tied or fenced at the time. Just then, Shanghai bounced around the corner wanting to play. Even though, just a puppy Shanghai stood almost 2ft. tall and Pete just brushing 2ft. himself was terrified of Shanghai. As any caring mother would do, without thinking of my stitches and stapling, I reached down and scooped my crying child up. Later that night, I realized why the no lifting instructions were so important, as I have done all a week now I'm proceeding to change my bandages and discover that I have succeeded in reopening the outer layer of my incision. No more bikini bathing suits for this now deformed body. You know sometimes somethings we've been told for our own good goes in one ear and out the other just like we never heard it. You know at 17 or any of the teenage year you tend to think no further than dinner and remember nothing passed breakfast I missed so many days from school while being sick and recuperating that if I'd missed one more I would've been kicked out for truancy. Still very sore I returned on the 15th and final day. While I was in the hospital during this ordeal I realized that Willie still cared because he brought me a stuffed brown German Shepard puppy. It was his sweet side that kept me dangling, wishing, hoping and crying because I wanted to hear him say "I love you" to me again. Although every fiber of my being 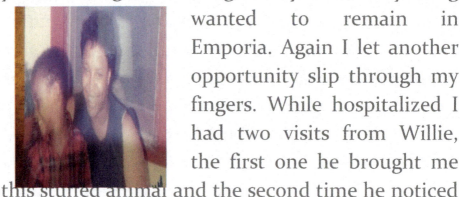 wanted to remain in Emporia. Again I let another opportunity slip through my fingers. While hospitalized I had two visits from Willie, the first one he brought me this stuffed animal and the second time he noticed I had written everyone's name that had visited but became angry that I had made his cousin's initials bigger than his. Neither one of us discussed the events that led up to this point. Sometimes when things go unsaid there's a silence that should not reign supreme. He was under Barbara Walker's delusions. I didn't know the full lengths she had gone to keep us apart until way too late. He had been coming around until he realized I had written his cousin's name bigger than his on the bottom of the dog. Really dude! Patches was my childhood road-dog but I loved you! Advocating for myself was never my strongest trait. Maybe that's why I losthim anyway. Neither one of us were very assertive back then. There's always been a certain kind of chemistry between us, it's electric, even right 'til this day. I can still look at him and melt. He is the only man that can read my every thought just by looking at me. Just hoping that I would get that second chance to love him again. Now that I'm paralyzed it's probably just a pipe dream, or on the other hand, if it does it's meant to be. As I attempt to get back on course with the story at hand, I've been back in Charlottesville for about six weeks and visit my OB/GYN for a regular check-up to find out that I have some abnormal cells on my cervix. A biopsy showed pre-cancerous tendencies. After meeting with the head OB/GYN doctor the recommendation was to have the cells frozen off and they would then be expelled naturally with my period which was brought on with oral stimulant pills. The freezing procedure was fairly easy with some expected pain. The period stimulant medicine made it feel as though I was back in labor and made me bleed profusely for two weeks. Again I would have to take iron supplements. Who knew having a baby could set off so many illnesses in a woman's body. It seems as if I've been falling apart since I gave birth. While everything else has me sidelined the dentist wanted his turn, I was informed that my wisdom teeth were impacted and needed to be removed. So I found out on a Monday and had surgery on Wednesday. On my way to the appointment we had to stop for gas, so when I went inside the store to pay, I spotted my favorite candy bar a Baby Ruth. Since I hadn't eaten since dinner, I just knew I'd be able to enjoy it after leaving the dentist office. Little did I know, my face was going to be swollen like a chipmunk with both cheeks packed with nuts. I was also black and blue. That candy bar remained unopened on my dresser for six weeks.

Whatever made a person that tripped going upstairs after returning from the dentist, think that they could be coordinated enough to ride a skateboard. Well leave it to me, I thought just that. Back in the 80s the mode of travel for a teenager was a skate board. Granted, I couldn't keep my balance on roller skates, so again I say why did I think I was coordinated enough to ride a skateboard? Still fairly new to Charlottesville and trying to make new friends I tried to be one of the in crowd. I wasn't stupid enough to go out and buy my own skateboard, but I liked to practice on my friends. They usually didn't mind, because they knew they would get a laugh out of it. The street that I lived on was on a hill that dead-ended into a parking lot that was surrounded by trees on three sides and a drop-off at the very back end of the lot. This parking lot usually was empty on the weekends, except this was the weekend of the Dogwood Festival Parade. Many people seeking parking that was free and close to the downtown mall, sought out this parking lot. But to teenagers that couldn't care about the parade, this street was the perfect place to learn how to skateboard. This street was on such a slope that if you got the right momentum at the top of the street you could ride it all the way down and back without any foot power at all. A policeman once clocked someone doing 45 mph downhill and the same person doing 20 miles per hour on the way back. Needless to say that person was not me. The one and only time that I've tried to ride the whole road, was going good until I hit the parking lot and tried to make the turn and come back up. Concentrating so hard on not going over the cliff, I never saw someone opening a car door. I managed to not wipe out or hit their car that second, but in maneuvering around them I lost my balance, slipped off the board, and the board went airborne and came down and scrape the side of another car. I didn't fall when I slipped off the board but as the board was coming down I got hit in the stomach and it dropped me to my knees. The skateboard twisting and turning as it fell scraped what looked like a 3 foot long gash into someone's passenger side. This was my one and only accident on a skateboard because I never got back on one.

Now that I don't look like Chip or Dale anymore, I'm on my way back to work at McDonald's. I've got staff telling me in my journal that I should look into jobs where I could use my training. One part of me knows that they're right, but the other part is trying to resist adulthood as long as possible. I got paired with Matilda Timberlake through the big brother and big sister program, thankfully her visits fall under therapy so I can still go on an outing. Remember how earlier I said it was easy to lose your level. Well, fighting is one of those things that results in immediate loss of every privilege you can think of: loss of free time, loss of phone privileges, loss of allowance and loss of 1 level. No matter the reason to staff if you fight with another resident the consequences are the same. In my defense, I never laid a hand on Mary although she deserved a good old country stomping. Have you ever known someone that just seem to exist solely just to piss you off? That was Mary W. to everyone else in the house, down to the little timid Angel who was afraid of getting out of bed most days. Mary would get right up in your personal bubble as if she had no clue that she was too close and spout something inappropriate about your family usually a mother comment. Those didn't usually bother me, but I would see red behind the racial and female dog bashing. That night Mary was in rare form. Still not in perfect health I just wanted to be left alone. It's a Friday evening about 7:05 Wheel of Fortune had just come on and I was comfortably planted in front of the air conditioner and TV. It was very obvious to everyone else that I was watching this program but apparently, she requested the television at 7, which wouldn't have been a problem if she'd just asked. Doing things the right way was always a stretch for Mary. Anyway when Mary jumped in my space I jumped back, and doused her with a brand new bottle of lotion from head to toe. Like a baby she cried out for staff. Because what I did was deemed an act of aggression I immediately lost my level 3 status and had to move back upstairs. I hate to have to move back into a room with another person, but it was worth the loss to get my point across. The other residents did not want to impose any kind of consequences because they applauded my action and wished I had beat her to death's door and back. I've never dealt with my personal space being invaded very well all my life or being called a bitch and these were Mary's top two go to offensives.

I've never been a bully but after standing up to Tammy in the 4th grade I learned to spot them. I also swore to never be intimidated ever again by another female. It was working until one Friday afternoon about dusky dark on Main Street I was walking uptown toward 10th Street pass A-1 car lot, the street lights had just come on. Have you ever had that eerie feeling that you were being followed? Well, unfortunately I have. That's terrible especially when it's true. I decided if a confrontation was going to happen this well- lit car lot would serve as the perfect backdrop, because it's right on the busiest part of Main Street near a cross street and a red light, so plenty of traffic should deter an unwanted attack. At least this was my mindset, unfortunately no one told the dike that chased me around for 5 minutes until I knew that my only choice was to fight. I have always been straight with no desire to bat from the left side of the plate, no one told her that either. When I inquired "why are you bothering me?" she replied "you have something I want." I offered my purse and all $57 that was contained within and pleas to be left alone went unheard. She panted and salivated as if I was prime rib on a salad bar. She held me pinned to a white Bonneville with her left hand around my throat and undid my jean zipper with her right. Just as she plunged her fingers in between my labia I managed to scream STOP just as the police car pulled up to the changing traffic light. By the Grace of GOD, my desperate cries were heard. The attack was thwarted, but not before making me feel violated. As the policeman drove me back to 7th Street he informed me that she had attempted to rape someone else in that very same car lot the past two weekends and they didn't handle the advances as well as I did. One ended up in the hospital with a broken eye socket and leg. The other one didn't survive. Who's to say I'm handling it fine? I'm shaking and jumping at every little sound. I have not gone anywhere by myself since. I can't continue being a hermit, or afraid anymore. After testifying against Cole in the judge's chamber because I'm still a few months away from 18, I realized I had to take back my composure, freedom and sanity. Until this very moment I have never even spoken about that violation to anyone before or even spoken her name since.

Feeling cramped and ready to control my own destiny I inform Community Attention Group Extreme System (C.A.G.E.S) as I renamed the girls home. I have rented a room from Emma Jones on 11th Street, this is my first time on my own in Charlottesville. No rules except pay my $65 a month rent on time, clean behind myself, and be in before 11p.m. when she "fasten the door from the unsavory riffraff" in her own words. At least they were the expressed rules. The unwritten rules became expressed as I broke or badly bent them. Maybe being so strict on me was because of the mother in her but a mother figure was the last thing I wanted. So after 3 months I secured an efficiency at the Alcove Apartment complex. Culture shock to go from paying $65 a month to

$250 + utilities, freedom is beginning to be costly. If not for the $235 in social security that I used to frivolously spend on clothes, shoes, junk food and entertaining so called friends I would've been hurting. Still fresh in my mind every month when I cashed this check, my father's death in April of 1983. Playing grown up has caused another boneheaded decision while on my own. Because I would set out on my way to school just to end up back at home after leaving CATEC. In trying to maintain the apartment I had begun working two part-time jobs that didn't leave much time for sleeping. It became easier to justify my actions to the point that I quit going to school in May with one month and 3 days left until graduation, still hoping to keep the apartment. In my defense I took the GED exam and received my certificate two days before graduation. Still just not the same, because I had enough credits to graduate but the time that I missed after gall bladder surgery left me hours to complete attendance requirements. A letter explaining the absences from my doctor could have given me a passing grade and an early but deserved graduation. Had I done my due diligence and enquiries I would have found this out back then. I didn't really at that time really think as far in the future as I should have or maybe just wanting to handle everything myself by the seat of my hot in the ass pants instead of exploring all options. I took the ASVAB test and scored in the top five percentile of the whole United States but was told that I would have to give up custody of my son I chose not to join. Little did I know Barbara Walker had managed to do just this by lying and keeping the court date from me? I also fell into that unlucky gap where if my social worker had filed the necessary paperwork after my father's death immediately I could have qualified for payments until finishing college.

Being uninformed again caused me to panic and make that stupid decision in May after reading an informative letter from Social Security Administration telling me that my benefits would be terminated as of June 1, 1984, because I would be 18. I started seeing what I'd be losing not what I already had gained. So after only 1 year of unrealized freedom I asked to be taken back into the foal at Community Attention. Justification had to be determined. Thankfully GOD had already blessed me with the gift of gab, I was allowed to return because of my counselor and I convinced the board that I still could benefit from further counseling. This time I was determined to use this resource wisely. Now that I'm 18, the younger residents don't understand why I chose to voluntarily return to this program, sometimes I question my own motivation also. Self-preservation cannot be the only reason; well there's not wanting to assume adult responsibilities. The first time I opened up about the passing of my father and not attending his funeral, really made me wonder did I really want to revisit this old boneyard. Although I was still in Emporia at the time of his funeral. To still keep up the lie or not to have to mourn the only champion parent I had; I chose not to attend. Maybe I was afraid of dealing with my mother. Looking back now, I missed the perfect time to step back into the life that I was accustomed too. Nonetheless I was living my destiny. I hadn't been gone long enough to lose my hatred for journals, but I understood their importance better. Staff noticed the change in my more mature attitude and writing style. Maturity is an overrated sentiment used by old people to make getting old sound enjoyable. I was coasting along working harder to understand the things that make me tick. Again staff has started bugging me about finding a job that utilizes my training, so my new challenge is to put in at least two applications for a certified nursing position in every day I have off. I have no idea why I have not tried to get a job in my field of training. An avoidance of responsibilities may be my biggest motivator. Adulthood terrifies me for some reason. Although I entered adulthood at 16, this group home placement has allowed me to regress for a bit. Finding out that the real world doesn't care about your apprehensions, does nothing to bolster your confidence.

I found out that Eldercare Gardens wants to interview me for a certified nursing position, I should be a shoo-in because I've been volunteering there for almost six months. I earned my certification before leaving Emporia. This is the single best thing I've done for my future employment endeavors. I went to work there September 1985 and worked morning shift supposedly, at least that's the shift I was hired for. Being young and having relatively no life I was free to work as much over time as I wanted. Having to report to work at 6:45a.m proved to be an impossible task that met with opposition immediately with co-workers. I had to catch the bus to work Monday through Friday which didn't get me there until 7:05. I did better on the weekends because the cab usually got me there on time, especially after I made a standing appointment with Yellow Cab Company. Eldercare Gardens like most nursing homes always had a shortage of reliable help especially on the weekends. Unfortunately, when you have a big heart or just have problems saying NO, maybe even unintentionally the "higher-ups" would overwork the dedicated ones. It is here that I learned about cliques in the workplace and social hierarchy. No matter how dedicated you are, if the leader of the pack feels threatened, your job is in jeopardy. I witnessed an incident of abuse well, neglect. Sometimes your patient load would be overwhelming, but you were expected to give the same quality of care whether you had 5 or 15. So often people will forget to leave their attitudes and problems outside of the workplace. I understand that this is a tough thing to do quite frequently. This particular day one of the Buckingham crew was having issues with her husband and quite frankly should have called in. Nonetheless she brought her problems and attitude to work. Sometimes when there's a patient that needs assistance and it's your lunch time things need to be prioritized. Well I think someone having to use the restroom should take precedence over your Bologna and Cheese, but who am I? Especially if that person has been screaming "Please, Please I got to go to the bathroom" for at least 30 minutes. Granted, this was an extremely busy day because we each had 15 patients. Nonetheless, what happened next should never happen, upon returning from lunch she discovered that her patient had used the bathroom in her pants and was sobbing, no fault of the patient because she was wheelchair confined. As the attendant wheeled the patient into her room, I overheard that aide cursing the patient out because she now needed to be bathed or showered and she also needed to clean her wheelchair. No one enjoys extra work, but this was avoidable. I offered my assistance, maybe to defuse the growing situation. I never wanted to cause any tension between us, but that is exactly what happened. Because that person knew she had done wrong, she decided to turn the story around and I became the abusive attendant in her version. She enlisted the help of her car mates, even though the charge nurse of the unit knew the truth, the director of nursing still fired me. I was told later that those women got away with lots of things because so many rode together so if they fired 1 they were risking losing 5 more. I was expendable, never mind patient rights.

Sometimes blessings happen when you're not expecting them. Well for months now I've been getting sick at different hours of the day, but not every day. Never in a million years would being pregnant have crossed my mind because I never missed a menstrual cycle. Looks like adulthood has caught up with me yet again. Too many cab rides from car 40. Time to start looking for an apartment. The staff agreed to let me stay until I found affordable housing or until the others figured out that I was pregnant. By the grace of GOD I found a job at Rose's Department store three days after leaving Eldercare Gardens. Finding an apartment proved to be more challenging. Word of mouth played a big part in me finding the cottage on Riverdale. At $250 a month I was set or so I thought, three months later my landlord sold the properties to the Shelter for Help in Emergency (S.H.E).

I still stayed in counseling with my counselor from the group home and kept my relationship with my big sister. Good thinking because I needed someone or something to keep me sane. Here I was right back at point 0, with zero leads and zero dollars for a second deposit in less than six months. My big sister was the coolest adult I knew and any advice, knowledge or wisdom she shared wasn't preachy, accusatorially or given as condemnation. She always helped me to evaluate every situation by the pros and cons. Maybe because she was the baby of three sisters or maybe because her parents were just as sweet, laidback, level headed and loving. Because they accepted me and welcomed me as if I was daughter number 4. Tilly was every kind of woman I wanted to become: successful, pretty, nice and independent. She only had one flaw that I could see, too demure—the ultimate Christian woman; no street moxie. It worked for her though because she had it all, the perfect job straight out of high school, a brand new car every 3 years, her own townhouse and a supportive boyfriend who was also a professional from a prominent local family. Tilly wanted to help take my mind off of my problem so she told me to be ready early that Saturday morning and wear comfortable shoes. She called at 7:00 a.m. and we met at Golden Skillet at 8:45 for breakfast or so I thought. Upon arrival she rolled down the window and said "get in." After getting in the car she said "We both can use a break so let's blow this city for the day." After we were on 64 for a while and some light conversation she asked "how's Kings Dominion sound?" I wasn't expecting that or even thinking about my birthday. So much had been happening that the calendar had sped past and now it's June 5, 1985. Once we hit Doswell we realized it would be cheaper to eat before we entered the park, so we went to Burger King across the street from the theme park. By that time it's now 10:30 and change over time—breakfast is ending. When we entered the restaurant the lobby was empty. The cashier had her back to the counter but said over her shoulder "I'll be with you in one minute". Because we didn't know what we really wanted this was okay. When the cashier turned around it was uncanny as if I was looking in a mirror even down to her glasses and hair style. Her name was Pam--- she was two years younger than me. She could have been my long lost sister.

Back to the old drawing board! June to September I saved every penny possible for a deposit and first month's rent. Everything out there was so expensive. A friend suggested becoming roommates. This should have been perfect except my money was about to change. So I came up with a solution, the first 3 months I'll pay the rent + utilities which is October through December and he was supposed to cover January through March. All should be good right, wrong, how did I miss his obvious drinking problem? Unfortunately I missed obvious signs that he had deeper feelings than I did also. Apparently while I thought we were just friends hanging out after work, (he-he-ha-ha) having fun, killing time with other co-workers. Or having a drink and going our separate ways for a couple years now, without as much as that oops I'm sorry I didn't mean to touch your ass, obvious feel. When I moved to the cottage something totally different must have developed in his mind. Even though he knows I'm expecting another man's baby. After further discussions he swears that we will just take things slowly. I foolishly believed that this conversation was over. We had found an apartment on short Caroline. Things seemed truly okay until Thanksgiving weekend. Friday night George came home drunk and crying. Never before had he blamed me of betrayal or using him, but these were his claims now. I'm praying for the precise words not to anger him further. After two crazy hours, he has fallen asleep. My hope for the night is for him to just sleep it off because I have to work tomorrow. No such luck, I can hear noises in the kitchen, hopefully he'll realize what he did earlier terrified me and did nothing for his positioning. I never thought that things would end up this way with this situation of convenience, my child is due in 1 month. My child's father has proven useless, so I now know I'm alone with whatever choices I have to make. I know also that I don't have funds to move again and I don't have the energy to continue trying to stay here either. Realizing it's quiet again, maybe I will be able to sleep for a few hours and attack this problem after work. I so hate sharing my business with anyone but I feel like if my supervisor was abreast of my situation, maybe she could advise me of how to terminate my lease without losing my money and my life. I finally made it through the longest Saturday of my existence. Having very little sleep and dealing with the after Thanksgiving shoppers for twelve hours, I'm beat. Being in my eighth month of this pregnancy, these marathon work schedules are starting to take a toll. But I need to accrue as much overtime as possible these last weeks, however many I can manage to squeeze in. The due date is predicted to be Christmas again and I was two weeks early with the other one. Praying for a few hours of uninterrupted solitude once I have finished this long walk home. On the weekend the bus schedules are modified on some routes. Luckily, since I've been working twelve hours on

Saturdays, I have had my Sundays free. Thanking GOD because it would be a struggle and expensive, the buses don't run here on Sundays.

I arrived home after walking what seemed to be five miles, to my aching feet and melt into my comfortably plush twin bed. Dinner will have to wait until I have had a well needed nap. Thankfully, it is as I like it, quiet, George wasn't home. I'm awakened by George at 11:45, he started with an apology and my keys, which I apparently left hanging in the deadbolt on the front door. Whew! Finally that craziness is over, at least I hoped. Monday, December 1st at my doctor's appointment I was informed that I was going to require a C section in order to deliver my baby, so I needed to choose which day to deliver. My choices were the 23rd or the 26th, because they don't schedule surgeries on the holidays. Tired of carrying this baby, I chose the earliest possible date. This news takes the worry off my mind and gives me a somewhat sense of the immediate future. I can inform everyone that will be interested, need to know or will be impacted. I told my mom as soon as I got home I also called Pete and his grandmother on his dad's side, and I attempted to reach this baby's father to no avail.

The one notification I wasn't looking forward to making came about 7:30 that evening. Knowing that I was definitely going to be sidelined for at least six weeks, I needed to know everyone was on board with all that was about to happen. I also wanted to feel the vibes I was receiving from everyone. Talk is cheap, actions speak the loudest. I haven't heard that very much from the baby's father this whole pregnancy, I can understand why George could feel like the stand in. Always on the go, I stay tired with this pregnancy, knowing I have to be at work bright and early, I turn in at 9. I don't even remember eating dinner.

I'm awoken at midnight by the stereo blaring. "Not tonight please!" I screamed as I turned the corner into the living room. George and his best friend are still on their Thanksgiving break from UVA maintenance. Usually I wouldn't mind if they hung out but unfortunately I've got to be up in five hours for work and giving the bombshell George hit me with during his last alcohol consumptive episode, I'd rather avoid this potential disaster. Do I stay and try to courteously waltz Henry and the liquor bottle toward the front door, risking the entanglement of feelings again or do I just let the night unfold as it may? I chose the latter, taking both guys at their word they would keep the noise down. It doesn't take me long to fall back to sleep only to be awakened again with George laying on my bed rubbing my belly. Normally this would not worry me, because he is a tender, caring soul. I didn't want to seem uncomfortable but I was nervous, I didn't want to anger him, I've only seen him cry once before, when his father died. I pretended to have to go to the bathroom in order to put some space between us safely. When I had pulled myself together I went into the kitchen for some water just to be cornered by my weeping roommate begging me to marry him and forget about the father of my baby. When I tried to let him off the hook easy, he changed into the scorned <u>lover</u>, I want to use that term loosely. Reasoning with him was out of the picture. He truly seemed angered, angry to the point that he tried to reinforce his position by threatening to harm one of us with his .25 caliber hand gun which was in his pocket, I felt it when he hugged me in the bedroom before I went into the bathroom. Keeping him calm was one thing on my mind at that time, keeping his hand out of his pocket was another. Putting him to sleep was the necessary evil at hand. Unfortunately back then I only knew one surefire way to put a man to sleep, sex. That wasn't something I wanted to do, but I wanted sleep. I knew that crossing that line sent a conflicting message more than all the messages before. Until now we have flirted around the idea of a real relationship not just the friends with benefits situation we have now. I have thought before about taking our relationship further but never wanted to lose the friendship. That friendship had been damaged, so why sex? A parting gift, just what I needed. Too much sexual tension pinned up for months. George was the type of man I was drawn to chestnut complexion, tall, slender, and easy on the eyes. He has the full package, usually I like the vibes between us but, his drinking seems uncontrollable. I'm not sure if the increased drinking was there and I never noticed or if it's increasingly been getting worse since we moved in together. Everything else about us in very good, he's very gentle and takes directions in the bedroom so well. I especially love the way he doesn't mind snuggling for hours. Most nights so I could fall asleep we would spoon until I drifted off to sleep, he was a source of comfort usually. I've seen him through two failed relationships and he has seen me through as many too. Why did things have to change so drastically this weekend? Maybe Wednesday will bring back the status quo, when he returns to work.

Wednesday, Thursday, and Friday were enjoyable, not only did George return to work, he started AA meetings. Although I am proud of the gesture, I know that things will prove one way or the other by Monday. Two days with nothing like work to occupy his hours away from me, not that I'm the "be all and end all" or anything. I know that free time is definitely the devil's playground. So many times before I've witnessed valiant efforts of a drinker fall desperately unfulfilled. Hoping and praying that George will not be just another black man that succumbs to a statistical downfall. To try to make it George rids the apartment of all liquor bottles. Was I that blind? All totaled there were 8 bottles scattered around this two bedroom apartment, one for every room and closet under the roof. How did I miss the signs? Especially since I saw this man almost daily for the past three years. Was I so enchanted by his infectious smile, humor, or love making that I couldn't see the forest for the trees?

Never get too comfortable things can change quickly. Paydays always brought on impromptu partying. My first stop is always the grocery store but George is struggling with changing his payday routines. Although we went grocery shopping together we usually have different ideas about what is cart worthy. We had decided that $35 per person would cover breakfasts and dinners for a month, because I got WIC (Women, Infants & Children) checks that covered milk, cheese and juices. Also because I received food stamps, George would give me his grocery money, because $35 in food stamps went further than straight cash. Nonetheless, we'd have arguments over beer, cigarettes and laundry detergent, which weren't covered. I've got our cart and I'm next in line, I don't see George anywhere, which could mean nothing or everything. Nothing could mean he's truly refraining from alcohol or he could be outside downing a forty right now. It's hard not being able to trust your roommate, lover or your own instincts. Time will tell. His next challenging moments will come in a few hours when he goes to his mother's house on Prospect Avenue alone, because when we have finished running errands for home, he'd help her on Friday evenings. He usually invites me along but lately I relish my time alone. Plus I'm not going to be able to protect him from himself if he really wants to drink. Anyway after working 12 hours 5a-5p today, all I want now is sleep. Either I budgeted better or $70 goes further without George over my shoulder, because there seems to be a ton of groceries to put away. A bologna and cheese sandwich with lettuce and tomato is all I've been craving all day. Good thing because that's all the energy I've got left. I'm too tired to care about having to fall asleep alone. In the cab ride home, we were both quiet and in neutral corners, I don't even know if we said 10 words since leaving Safeway. George jumped right back into the cab after unloading the groceries.

Sleep is a commodity to a pregnant woman. An interruption of said sleep should be a punishable criminal act. It's 2a.m. and George has fallen off that proverbial wagon, I know because that is the only time he wanted to blast music. Usually he was quiet and laidback. Unfortunately as of late he's an instant asshole just add alcohol, a crying drunk nonetheless. I don't do well with crying adults if it isn't about an injury or a death, everything else can be worked through. Tears don't make anyone empathetic to alcoholics, at least not me, especially not when I'm sleepy. Deal with it so I can go back to sleep, is my thought. Entering the living room with a different approach, "Baby we got to work in 4 hours, let's go to ...." Before I could finish the sentence, I heard the gun being cocked. Thankfully he didn't look up as I entered. I ran back to my room, grabbed the phone, I ran into his room, hid in the closet and called 911. I had no idea what state of mind he was in, but the police could find out and deal with him. Its December 6th 2:45a.m. The police dispatcher stayed on the phone with me until the officers got me safely out of the back bedroom window. As I was climbing out of the window, I could hear another officer talking to George. So the Lord saved my life and maybe even George's that morning.

That was scary! The police took me to my big sister's house. I was shaking like a leaf, but after telling my ordeal, I fell asleep on her couch. Eight o'clock came way too soon. My sister loaned me an outfit and shoes so I could go to work. When I got there I guess the reality of what I had gone through set in and I also realized I hadn't felt my baby move since the previous day, now I'm worried. I called my supervisor over to my register and asked if I could leave to go to the hospital to make sure my baby was alright. While at the Emergency room I had to repeat my story several times but that was okay because they referred me to the SHE shelter. This wasn't the way I would have chosen to get out of my lease, but it worked. Fortunately my placement in this program isn't temporary, so I will have somewhere to return to after I deliver. At least I will have a little time to work out my situation. When I returned to work on Tuesday the 9th there seemed to be a huge burden lifted. Back in another setting that requires you to examine your feelings; at least this time I understand myself better and realize how grateful I am for God's grace and mercy. Because of the ordeal and late stage of my pregnancy I decided to quit working twelve hours every day and made the 20th my last day until the New Year.

At the doctor's appointment on the 22nd I had to sign all of the "pre-admit paper "work, for that night's admission. I checked in after 7p.m. Although the C section is scheduled for tomorrow, the time isn't. If there are no emergencies, my surgery will be early in the morning. I'm nervous surely but excited also. My baby girl will be here inside of fourteen hours. I was hoping to be going home to my own apartment, but this maybe is going to be better because I won't be totally alone, in case something happens, not that I think it will. I hope to get some sleep tonight because it probably will be the last for a while. I still need to find the same things I was searching for after my first pregnancy: childcare, housing and the money to afford both. Rose's pays decent, but I still would need to find a place for $250-$300 a month, so much for wishing. Right now all I can pray for is a healthy baby.

It's almost 1:30p.m.and my stomach feels like its touching my spine, because of surgery I've been NPO since midnight, ice chips only tease a stomach. The nurse has told me I was next, I should be spoiling my baby girl by 3:45. That made me smile and giggle. Although giddiness was all over my face, a small part of me still longed for freedom, or at least for my mother helicoptering as she did when Pete was born. This time I was all alone, I was hoping Charles the baby's father would have been here, but he chose to work, or at least that was the excuse of the day. Lately I've been getting more excuses than enough. I've known for almost the whole pregnancy that I would be on my own because he wanted me to abort the pregnancy from the moment I told him. Katherine his older on again off again girlfriend, works here at UVA and had to make her presence known earlier this morning. She knew I was here, I guess Charles informed her or maybe she positioned herself in such that she would transport my roommates back and forth, she has already been in my four bed ward 3 times since 8:00a.m. As a member of the transportation team, she had every right to be in maternity unit, so why pretend. Pretending she didn't know I was there, that she was concerned and cared. Nonetheless she never even spoke directly to me. I was the one that stood between her and happiness. Knowing that although distant now Charles will come around once this baby is born. She still felt threatened by my being able to give him a child. Silly though because they both have children from other relationships. Her children were almost adults and his daughter was at least seven. I and my child should not have been any kind of threat. I think she just wanted to intimidate me but nothing was going to make me worry that day. At least not another human being except my baby.

It's finally time to be moved to the surgical holding room. The closer I get to the operating room, the more the nerve's take over. Am I really ready, nonetheless its happening? My last birthday I turned twenty, now six months later, I have only minutes left to cling to anything called youth.

Grown-up tears welled up behind my eyes when the nurse told me it was time to get an epidural, already getting nervous, with that news anxiety just became terror. I remember singing that Oh so familiar song "It's me again Lord" trying to not think about the medical team inserting an IV into my spine. Putting complete trust in the Almighty surgeon Jesus and believing he would guide the anesthesiologist's hand and obstetrician who was delivering my child as soon as the numbing cocktail has finished running in. I'm feeling drowsy but trying hard not to fall asleep. Just as the nurse predicted its 3:45 and I'm holding my 9lb. 6oz., curly head, 10 perfect fingers, 10 perfect toes, and lighter walnut complexioned huge BOY! YES, again the predictions missed the mark, I just needed to hear the doctors say he was healthy. At first glance the pediatrician thought he had megalocephaly I think I learned the true meaning of prayers throughout the next 48 hours because the pediatric neurologist was having him tested every few hours. One by one every examination, every X-ray, and every tube of blood proved that GOD takes care of young children. Demetrice was given a clean bill of health on Christmas around dinner time. On Christmas the women's auxiliary volunteers would knit red or green stocking caps for every baby in the nursery and put your baby in a Christmas stocking, my baby was too big to fit either, so they fashioned him a stocking cap out of IV protectant gauze and placed his Christmas stocking in his crib near his feet. The sentiment was still accepted. I was grateful he was alive, healthy and normal. Now that he was here, I had bigger worries, where were we going to live? By the time we were discharged it was New Year's Eve.

Back at the shelter, I discovered that personal belongs left in an empty bedroom for a week became public domain. I was in no position to fight for articles of clothing or shoes. Staff of course asked the residents to return anything they had taken, but no one seemed to know anything. Adulthood will grow you up fast. Immediately I went from being prepared for a newborn to needing everything except formula, only because the hospital gave me enough to last until I could get my baby registered for WIC. I only have the diaper bag I had bought from a handcrafting expo because I took it with me to the hospital. What a way to start a new year. Nonetheless my baby needed me to be stronger than I've ever been. Focusing on finding an apartment was of the utmost importance, looking in the classified advertisements was yielding no results, for over a week and a half, I started to panic. On January 12th a lady that needed a live-in nanny called and enquired about help with 3 daughters. Word to the Wise: Never say never! Desperation will make you climb down from your pedestal and do what is necessary versus what is comfortable. The staff knew Miss Jane because she too had once sought refuge at this very shelter from an abusive husband. With a recommendation from my counselor, I gave it a chance.

My first evening on top of the mountain was spent meeting the girls, hearing Jane's wishes and cleaning the bedroom, so I would have a place to lay my head. Clearing a year's worth of unworn, too small clothing that the family had forgotten about or couldn't find matches too. The family was reeling from a divorce. The mother was throwing herself into work and the father become MIA. The girls have been fending for themselves for about six months, and the house reflects it all. Mary Poppins I'm not but hoping this will be as good for me as them. Jane works evenings at a nursing home and sleeps until one hour before work, so I have the house to myself 75% of the time, which is good because the house required so much attention, someone under foot would get on my nerves. A maid would have hated taking this job, I keep reminding myself that it's a place to live for the moment. It is far from free, but nothing has to come out of pocket except pampers and my toiletries. Thank GOD for somewhere safe, somewhere I don't have to worry whether my belongings are going to be where I left them, somewhere that my baby was not at risk of being bitten by a spider, rat, or another child. The youngest child here is in first grade, I think she's six. The girls are sweet but miss their parents, a stand-in isn't what they want, and I can totally understand this. I wondered how long it would be before the kids turned into little demons acting out for attention. Like a lot of divorced families when dad divorced mom he divorced the whole family. Unfortunate for the girls because the sun rose and set with their father. Jane used the children as bargaining chips. She once stepped into my room and admitted she didn't think I loved my son because she had never heard me tell him. Maybe she assumed I was like her, seeing dollar signs above his head, to her each child was worth $625per month because she received $2350 alimony and child support, with child support being the lion share. My WIC appointment was well appreciated, although I wasn't required to provide anything needed in house I feel better because I am able to contribute to the groceries. The extra milk, cereals, cheese, eggs, juices and peanut butter was a hit with the children because Jane had reduced them to bologna sandwiches for lunchtime, hotdog and beans for dinnertime, things the kids could prepare themselves in the microwave. Since I've been here we've had home cooked meals every night. Usually I would finish cooking before Jane went to work, she seemed happy to skip off with lunch in hand. I may not be kin but to give the resemblance of family to everyone seems to warm the mood of the house. Now that the girls have gotten use to me being around in the afternoons they look forward to an after school snack, or an early dinner and a bedtime snack. On top of the smiles this generates a bit of normalcy for the children. Jane even started emerging from her cave sooner and engaging me in conversation. She asked me "how have you been getting around since you don't have a driver's license or a car?" Not that she's ever tried to restrict my coming or going, she did tell me she expected me to be here every evening when the two youngest girls got off the school bus. I once thought she was spying on me when I came home ten minutes before the bus and still spent another 15 minutes in the cab. When I explained that I was talking to the baby's father, she told me he could visit anytime within reason. Little did I know that was going to be the beginning of the end, the very first time he visited she began walking around in skimpy night gowns and pretending she forgot he was visiting. Once can be forgiven, but only once, not every time. Since that was her house to avoid confrontations I asked Charles not to return to the house while she was home, I simply started looking for a new residence. Dealing with the girls was easy but Jane was a twisted pierce of work, one that I'd rather not put up with just for a free room.

Charles and I moved to Southwood trailer court. 87 Bitternut Lane was the second and last time to have a joint lease. I tried to do the "home body", wife like things to let him take care of us for two months until he left me stranded without pampers and milk. Having a godmother for Demetrice was supposed to mean that she'd provide for my son in case something happened to us (his parents) not because we were not caring for him. I felt like a failure when I had to call her. I made my big sister Tilly his god mother. I decided at that very moment never to depend on anyone else to take care of me or my son. I found a job, a babysitter and made sure my child never went without again. I continued to stay in this trailer until the county housing certificate became available. Walking from Southwood to Fifth Street Food Lion and back to make a home for us.

My own affordable apartment at Whitewood Village became available in September 1987, I had never been so happy to do a walk through. Finding out that this apartment had two bedrooms and laundry machines downstairs, I was set. When we moved in on October 4th everything I owned fit into the back of a station wagon cab. I had clothing for both of us, his crib, stroller, high chair, play pen, walker and a voucher for furniture from the Salvation Army. With that voucher I found living, dining and bedroom furniture, of course used but brand new to me. Having tried to be a good homemaker in Southwood I had kitchen stuff, linens and towels. It felt good to tuck my baby in, in his own room that didn't have a hole in the floor that you could see the grass and critters that dwell beneath. This apartment was the best place I have ever lived alone as the only adult, the one in charge. No one looking over my shoulder, no one to impose a bedtime or curfew. No one to object to my smoking in front of my TV. No one except my baby and myself to pick up behind. I also noticed the quiet after a night. I never before had the deal with the noises of neighbors everywhere—above me walking like giants, below me knocking on the ceiling when I vacuumed too loud or too long. My bedroom was right against the stairs and every footstep echoed and every voice from the hallway sounded amplified but muffled.

Although the apartment was ours, the solitude was unbearable. I asked my little sister to come stay with us for selfish reasons I think but anyway she agreed. I needed a baby sitter and someone to talk to or argue with. Have you ever regretted a decision as soon as it was executed? Living with someone under staff supervision isn't the same when you're in charge. Especially if you don't know how to discipline yourself. Realizing that people can be trifling and undisciplined when left to be adult-like. I didn't take into account the way we met, at the group home and how I became her big sister. I was roped into the title by a user. I didn't recognize this at the beginning, the first time I left the girl's home I was a means of convenience. I became her scapegoat anytime she wanted to leave for a long period of time when she wasn't allowed privileges. I would receive a phone call at work asking if we could hang out after group meeting on Mondays. Usually she just wanted to hook up with her boyfriend and needed an exit strategy. Nonetheless I needed child care. So the second bedroom became her domain to live as she chose too. As long as she cared for my son while I worked. Once that became too much to expect of her, I began looking for daycare outside the house and applied for help from Social Service. I asked Missy to move out and had to fumigate that bedroom from top to bottom. I never knew that a female could be so trifling.

The location of this apartment posed challenges in getting to work especially on Sundays. Still too new to request every Sunday off, catching a cab should be free but not. Since I chose to move Charles decided to marry his on again off again girlfriend Katherine, that wedding announcement appeared in the paper one week after my move. I'm not jealous because I got the better part of that deal without the chains of marriage. There's nothing better than realizing that GOD protects children and fools. Since I'm was looking forward to celebrating my 22nd birthday next, I guess I'm the latter. Just for a quick change, I took a job at Giant. It's closer to home and pays the same as Food Lion. The position will definitely be temporary because I applied for the cashier or stock position, but the only immediate opening they had was in the salad bar. So I had to accept it of course, just to avoid a break in paychecks, but working in a refrigerated room every day is a chilling thought. Thank GOD for a good exit, I interviewed with Burger King again, this is always my fall back job. This will be my third time employed by Burger King and probably not my last. Had I stayed my first time, or even my second time back when I joined in high school, I could be a general manager by this time, but again I say hindsight is 20/20. Although I'm taking a cut in pay, the peace of mind is worth it. From the beginning I let them know that I could not work on Sundays. Usually this is a second job to bring in extra money for school shopping or Christmas but until I can do better, it's my primary job... I'll just have to figure out how to make $5.56 an hour pay the same bills that $7 was. I remember learning every way of enjoying noodles during this time because of course some kind of change in funds meant something went lacking. So any extra money that I saved from traveling back and forth across town to Food Lion I spent in daycare until I was approved for help from DSS. I changed jobs, loss the full-time status, and the difference in pay made my food stamp increase.

I also applied at UVA for a CNA position. I got my application in just before the summer freeze, so if not right away, I should be hired within 3 months. Although my time at Giant was relatively short, it left lasting memories, health issues, friends, enemies and stories. I was there six months, five and one half too many, because after I was passed over for transferring to the front or another department that needed cashiers three times, it became clear that I was stuck. Stuck because none of the people hired for the salad bar right before or after me was still working. That was the most grueling job I've ever held. I know now why butchers and chefs make so much, but exit the profession early because of health related issues such as arthritis, respiratory issues and or stress. Many people cannot work in cold conditions and I'm one of them. I realized that my productivity levels differ by 13%, with temperature variances of 5-10°. I like being able to feel my fingers, toes and not seeing every word I utter. It's hard to maintain sanitary conditions when your nose is so cold that it is running every day like you are suffering from allergies or a head cold with post nasal drip. I found out that cotton balls shoved up your nostrils help to keep your airway from totally drying out from the cold and aid in catching the drips. You have to invest in quality cotton balls, because of stray fibers or loosely packed fibers that could be accidentally inhaled. This I know first- hand because I suffered walking pneumonia while working there. I'm not sure if inhaling cotton fibers or if the constant temperature changes was the cause. Nonetheless, I had to leave. That's how and why I landed back at Burger King.

    After back at Burger King, it was about a month before I could make myself go into the walk-in refrigerator or the freezer without propping the doors opened. I don't think I had ever experienced claustrophobia before but each time I tried to retrieve anything from refrigeration I seem to have some sort of panic attack. The whole time behind those steel doors that entombed the cold or frozen inventory was nauseating. I could do any job required in the store blindfolded, but to count cold inventory I had to prop open all doors to the point that the temperatures would change about 3° by completion, because I would get winded, start breathing faster, start perspiring and get light headed and all. Possibly even though not still contagious I was still feeling remnants of the pneumonia. Nonetheless I was determined to make Burger King work until the perfect job opportunity became available.

The whole summer came and went before hearing anything from any position that I had applied for. I can only assume that the college students had scooped all worthwhile positions until time for classes to resume in the fall semester. I finally received an interview with UVA Health Services and I was hired as a certified nursing assistant. I was assigned to Barringer three. Barringer 3 was the cancer floor for adults. Everyone on this ward was in a life or death struggle with their bodies. Most of the patients have lead long, meaningful lives with some habits like drinking or smoking, those afflicted this way is understandable. But those that have lead healthy, clean living, exercising, eat right lives that still end up with an aggressive form of cancer overtaking more than one major organ, this is very hard to understand and except. It was brutally hard to deal with the passing of Mr. Roger C., he was a patient for most of his 17th year of life, other than being cured all this kid wanted was to live long enough to see his eighteenth birthday and he did just that. He was a fun loving, blond haired, blue eyed, true blue Redskins' fan. On any given Sunday evening you could hear far too loud cheering coming from room 7. Roger's whole family mom, dad, three brothers, two sisters, a gang of cousins, an aunt and two uncles would all be dressed in yellow isolation gowns, gloves, and hot face masks enduring hours of football from behind all that protective clothing just to watch the Redskins and any other game with Roger. The Saturday of Roger's birthday I wasn't scheduled to work but I traded nights with someone so I could give him his birthday present on his birthday. I didn't come in until 11p.m., Roger got his wish. He was born at 6:45p.m and he died two hours before I reported for duty. He never got to see the handcrafted Redskin throw that I got him for his birthday, I still gave it to his family who were still saying their goodbyes when I arrived at 11. I was so upset about this loss that I transferred to the emergency room.

My mother asked why the emergency room? In my mind it made sense to me. Yes I may encounter death, but I wouldn't have to watch the progressive deterioration of any one individual. In the emergency room you see people on their way to their next destination. The emergency department stay so busy that you never have time to mourn the losses or celebrate the achievements. When I was being trained my preceptor told me the emergency room motto was: "**Treat them and street them or bag them and tag them**". My first night of work I witnessed a doctor crack open the chest of a heart attack victim with a saw and I assisted the team while they massaged the heart back to sinus rhythm. The second night I made 7 trips to the blood bank in less than three hours. I loved it, the pace was bananas, the patients were interesting and I learned so much. It would have been the perfect place to work if everyone could work together as a team, six months in I found out that I was pregnant again, but with this one my doctor advised against lifting more than 10lbs, this time I was going to follow doctor's orders. Everyone that I worked with stated they understood the lifting restrictions but no one was ever able to give assistance when I needed it. So during my fifth month's examination I was given direct orders no lifting. When I delivered the news to my supervisor I was forced to leave because she said she could not guarantee me a position after I delivered and if I could not lift I would be handicapping the unit. Although she would not come out and say you're terminated. She gave me assignments that required lots of stocking, bending and lifting. I regretted giving her the satisfaction of winning but my baby's health and mine were more important than the job. Sitting home for five months wasn't as hard as I had anticipated. The baby's father and I have a cat and mouse relationship going on at best, we seem to be on different schedules all the way around especially since I have been working night shift at the hospital for over 11 months. Every now and again we find ourselves on the same page. We met when I worked at Giant, JC used to stop and carry on a conversation with me about anything for any amount of time. We could make each other laugh no matter the prior mood. The conversation could range from witty banter to political, religious, philosophy or anything between. JC would give me rides home from work, maybe I really should have gotten a car of my own long before I did. The more we talked about nothing the better we got acquainted and the more he proved to be my type. You know that average boy next door type, the one that doesn't readily stand out but slowly worms his way to that place in your heart. When you realize on your day off that there is something missing, but you can't quite place what it is, that's him. We could have been something special for a great period of time if not for alcohol and other habits. At least this time I could recognize the pattern. As funny as JC is, I can't trust that things will work out. JC tried to put on straight faces whenever I saw him. JC would come by less frequently after I lost the job at UVA. I decided not to push the issue.

I started walking to my girlfriend Liz's house almost every day just to get out and to get exercise. This one Friday evening her whole family was there. I had already met her mom and dad beforehand but never her brothers or nieces. I tried to excuse myself but one of the brothers locked on and started asking a million questions. He was a character, interesting. Totally different from my usual type stocky, lighter walnut complexion, less than six feet tall and soft. Well maybe not soft but not a thug by far. Emmett was different in other ways also he hated a paycheck, he liked money but not holding down a nine to five. He was comical, he was smart as a tack but spent more time trying to find the simple, easy, short cut from point A to point B. He could squeeze a dollar to death and spend a million on a square egg. He was different in the fact that he had custody of three of his daughters. Emmett came to visit me once before I had the baby, he cleaned my house and rearranged my furniture just as I instructed in exchange for me to wash and braid his three daughter's hair for the first week of school. I thought it was a win- win situation. This was the beginning of an interesting bartering relationship. All through August and most of September this was the standing agreement.

At 11:45p.m on September 27th, I had a very sharp pain cut across my back and it sent me running to the bathroom. My water didn't break but I started to spot and I made my way to the hospital, this time doctors got my predicted due date right. I wasn't going to take any unnecessary risk. Fortunately I didn't have to be placed on bed rest during this pregnancy, my doctor had warned me if I couldn't stop lifting that would be the next step to protect the fetus. The doctor was going to let me have this baby naturally since I've delivered both ways, but as my contractions got stronger, the baby's heart rate dropped. After being in labor overnight, Doctor Hill decided to do a C section about 1p.m. By the time they assembled a team, it was two when I was wheeled into the operating room and my baby Dameon was born on September 28th at 2:50p.m. Dameon was 7lbs 8oz and had a head full of curly black hair. Yet another healthy boy that had been predicted to be a girl. I had already decided to have my tubes tied after delivery, so I now have determined that I'm a boy factory and a girl is not in my DNA makeup. Also because this is going to be my last child I decided to breastfeed as long as possible. We were hospitalized for a week. When we finally made it home the little girls from next door met us at the top step screaming they wanted me to meet Dameon, although no discussion had happened, they had named their new pet goldfish Dameon too. I only came up with the name after laying eyes on him. Even though JC was in the delivery room choosing that name was all me. Many people asked if he was named for that kid from the movie <u>The Omen</u>, nope still to this day I haven't seen it.

    Time to regroup and figure out the future. No permanent position waiting for me, so I have six weeks to figure it out. Still in pain from surgery, I'm in no hurry yet. I know that I'll be working the polls on Election Day, that's as far in the future that I could see. Election Day was a month and 12 days away. Whoever babysits that day will have to be super trusted. I'm still breastfeeding and having problems trying to pump, so the babysitter will have to bring Dameon to DMV at least twice during that day, at least it's less than a mile away from Whitewood and Emmett did drive. So I did enlist the help of Emmett and company a few times before having to actually leave the boys for any great length of time. I can truly say Emmett loves children as much as I do and at least watching my children didn't qualify as work. The payoffs were worth it. Somewhere over the last weeks Emmett went from being my girlfriend's brother to being a person of great interest. Have you ever had to defend your domain against someone that had no clue? One Saturday morning Emmett's ex got bold enough to barge into my apartment as if she could regulate something. I was in my bedroom but I heard a strange voice speaking to the children. I know that the kids knew not to invite someone into the house that they didn't know. I rounded my bed to meet Pat in the hallway in front of the bathroom door. No one gave her the memo about pointing a finger in my face. She was yet another wannabe bully. If she'd acted as if she had the God given talent to talk to us as a concerned parent I would never have given her a swirly. YES the kind that nearly drowned her. Wait I'm sorry I just skipped straight to the end. Here's the full accounting.... She wanted to take her girls somewhere just to be ignorant. They wanted to stay with their older sisters. Which I could understand because during the week they all were scattered in different places. So my apartment and their aunt's was a peaceful sanctuary. She wasn't angry that they were with their dad but because they're near me. Why is it that the new woman is never good enough to be around your children? Well anyway I was seen as a mortal enemy no matter that I sent them home clean and happy. OOPS off on one of my tangents back to the story... After barging in unannounced she decided that a confrontation with me was the right next move. She was another one of those folks that couldn't seem to talk without pointing her finger in your face. After a warning to add insult to injury she fucked up and actually made connection with my nose. So I had no other options but to defend myself. I clapped down on that finger and didn't let go while punching her in the face hard and repeatedly. I have this thing about taking control of any fight because I fear being hit in the face. So I bit her finger so hard she lost the tip and half the nail. To polish her off I dunked her whole head into the toilet probably trying to kill her but I remembered the children in the other room.

A daycare is or had been in the back of my mind for a while now as potential work. I get bored so quick with being indoors, that would make me stir crazy, but it had to be given serious consideration because daycare is expensive. So this would solve two dilemmas, my own need of daycare and a job. I've been teetering on the brink of depression more this go around than with either one of the other pregnancies. I believe that having my life in turmoil the other two times didn't allow me time to stop long enough to realize the pain in my heart. Postpartum depression is a real condition that most don't get treated for, me included. Nine times out of ten someone suffering from it, doesn't recognize the symptoms. Or knowingly and intentionally skip seeking professional help, because of the label that society attaches to any type of mental illness. Different from baby blues, postpartum depression can continue for months and even years left untreated, I believe. I only became aware of what PPD was after my final pregnancy and realized I probably suffered from it with all three pregnancies. There's nothing worse than knowing that one of the happier times of your life feels like your loneliest and you can't shake this feeling. Maybe when I'm able to return to work I'll feel better is what I kept telling myself, I truly hoped. I never felt like hurting the boys but I had the overwhelming feeling that they would be better off without me. I don't remember how long those feelings lasted but I remember the day I decided to act on the feelings, I went to Food Lion and purchased 3 boxes of Unisom and dissolved them into a Coca-Cola and drank it. Had it not been for GOD's intervention by way of my next door neighbor wanting to borrow something, I would've been gone in January of 1990. I let feelings take over, instead of realizing that becoming a stepmom to 6 children ranging in ages from thirteen down to five without help in parenting from Emmett, the ultimate child. It was as if he wanted to be their friend and didn't enforce any rules. At those ages I had rules and chores. Because they didn't stay with us during the week he gave them freedom to come and go between my apartment and their aunt's place, which was okay until I cut into their plans trying to get their hair done before Sunday evening. Everyone wanted to be the last head done, because it had to last the whole week. No one wanted to get done on Friday evening, so I would spend most of Saturday washing clothes and hair and also braiding four girl's heads, at first it was fun, after a while it became expected. Especially after returning from the hospitalization I just didn't want to feel obligated. I also needed help with dealing with teenage angst.

Now along with having to navigate through the teenage hormones and mindset, I'm also having to try to assure JC and Charles that I'm well enough to care for our children. My hospitalization was used against me not because they feared for their child's safety, but I knew it was because they wanted to stop paying child support. For months each one filed different documents with Albemarle and Fluvanna County courts. Each court system awarded joint custody to the fathers with me having physical custody. Since the outcome wasn't as they had wanted withholding child support was their next move. I have seen friends go through the exact same thing, as if this was out of some throwback handbook written by yet another deadbeat dad, as if not paying $35 one week or every week for five months will make or break a good mother. Yes I may have struggled a little bit but I refused to beg them to provide anything.

I can understand why someone may have concerns about leaving children in the care of a person suffering from depression of any kind. I'm glad that you don't have to disclose any prior issues to become a daycare provider because I became a certified daycare provider for Charlottesville and Albemarle Social services in March of 1990. In order not to go stir crazy I also returned to PVCC part time. Like any business, starting a daycare took advertisements and patience, I seemed short on both. Right away I received two referrals from Albemarle social services but in order for that to be lucrative I needed at least two private pay children also. I gave it until June to prove profitable or else. Early into this adventure the children that were from social services their parents would not pay on time and I only had 1 private pay child that was going to be leaving in May. I still gave it until the beginning of May and since things weren't looking better, I decided to enroll in school full time starting in June. Irony would creep into play, no sooner than the following week after enrolling in school, social services wanted me to take 3 new children. I weighed my options and still chose school.

I applied for a work/study position but there wasn't anything available in my field at that time, so I threw all effort into finding a job that would work with my crazy school schedule. I found myself back at that old standby Burger King yet again. I say Thank GOD for good exits. I worked a three day weekend. Until school started I was able to work extra days during the week when I had a babysitter. I also applied for daycare assistance from social services which paid for daycare weekdays and provided bus passes. While I was pregnant with Dameon I took a semester towards office/administration and health procedures. With the passing years, four pregnancies and health issues; I'm finding that classes are much harder. When you're in high school you don't appreciate the simplicity of life. The ability to roll out of bed and shower and go. Now having to get two little ones bathed, dressed, fed and to daycare all before the door closes promptly at 9:46 in Senora Cook's beginners Spanish class. Three hours of conjugating verbs, constructing sentences and taking daily pop quizzes all before having breakfast can really tax a brain. Then feeling faint, confined and inadequately prepared, we were given thirty minutes to eat, prepare ourselves for one on one conversations with each other and/or the instructor. This was every Monday until 3, then to the learning lab for an hour. It was worse being in three different classes on Tuesdays and Thursdays from 10-4:45. That grueling schedule was 15 credits towards a degree that I never achieved. I used to joke that I was working on a twenty year plan for a two year degree. Looking back I know I wanted a means of putting food on the table and if an education happened along the way so be it.

A friend's challenge led to my next job. The challenge was to get my license and become a school bus driver. I failed the driving test twice using JC's car which I drove all the time. Frustrated about this I was showing it all over my face when I encountered my next door neighbor at the mailbox, after she laughed at me, she handed me her keys and said "go get that paper. " I did just that on the first try. Good thing too because the job listing was closing the next day. I received a call on Monday, interviewed Tuesday and started training on Wednesday. Karma or irony made me have to call my mother and apologize for an argument some years back, where I declared "I would never be like you ever." In order to provide for me better she had gone to school at night to get her CNA when I was 10, she already worked for a private family as a maid for many years and was in her 17th year as a school bus driver, now I've reached that moment in life where I realized I have become my mother and moreover I was proud of it. Proud of the get up and go work efforts that I learned from my mother. Proud that I could regroup and thankful that the Lord didn't allow me to remain in that dark place for long. Proud that God always provided the tenacity, the will and the opportunities to be self – sustainable; never needing to beg the fathers for help.

So, I had to tell her I'm sorry and get any advice or tips she could give me. I remember standing next to the driver's seat looking to the rear of the bus and realizing just how long of a vehicle I was about to start handling. I remembered how loud and rowdy children could be. I wondered was I really ready? Barely over the age of a high school student myself, now I'm going to be transporting Charlottesville's most precious cargo twice a day, Monday through Friday. My first assignment took me up and down streets that I've never traveled before, to neighborhoods that I didn't even know existed but it was fun. It's almost unfathomable to believe or to understand how a 40 foot long vehicle can handle as easy as a Volkswagen bug. My mom used to say that because you are sitting so far above others, it's easy to see 360° which makes it easier to maneuver. You just have to be always on alert for craziness from the others on the road around you. I now understand why Mom would take a few minutes to regroup after parking her school bus before jumping behind the wheel of her personal vehicle.

My mom had lots of stories to share about school bus antics but nothing stood out like this one: One Friday evening as we usually did, we crossed paths with my father, he would be returning from his last delivery to the paper mill in Roanoke Rapids North Carolina, which was just five miles across the state line at the end of the intersecting roads, a mile behind him. Usually he would ask if I wanted to get off the bus and go home with him and I would decline the offer, but that evening before he offered I was gathering my things and screaming mom can I go with dad as I saw him approaching the stop. Something seemed to compel me to say this. I'm convinced now that it was GOD's divine intervention because approximately twenty five minutes after I got off the bus my mom encountered a drunk driver on the narrow winding road that we lived on. Macedonia road is one of those country roads that had a series of curves that connected together like a snake. Combining a curvy narrow road, a speeding drunk and a school bus with a great defensive driver can still be the makings of a potentially deadly situation. The police said that had anyone unrestrained by a seatbelt been on the bus they would have died because the bus rolled over twice when trying to avoid the head-on collision. There was nowhere for mom to go, the shoulder on the right was a drop off and the left shoulder was a pond. She, being afraid of water, chose the drop-off. We were unaware of what had happened and that mom was involved, but we heard the crash over a mile and a half away. By the Grace of GOD, battered and bruised my mother walked away from the accident. Luckily another car was behind mom's bus because this was a time before cell phones. There's no telling how long it would've taken for someone to find her because the drunk driver fled the scene.

I couldn't drive a stick shift vehicle comfortably, every car before has been automatic. I constantly traded buses with other drivers being the newbie, I was hired as a relief driver, which meant I drove whatever route needed to be covered for however long. Each route had an assigned bus. In the fleet was four types of buses:

1. The flat nose Bluebird: By far the easiest to handle and most fun to drive. Looks like an orange transit CAT. This school bus is an automatic and the longest rig in the fleet.

2. The baby Bluebird: This school bus has all the bells and whistles of its longer big brother but has less regular seating to make room for up to four wheelchairs.
3. The regular Ford: This style was the oldest automatic in the fleet, most abundant, most unreliable and dare I say my favorite because of automatic and age. This model had only forty passenger seats.
4. The stick shift International: The original fleet. The five speed. The bane of my existence. The source of my terror. This vehicle had the best pulling power and was the best on gas.

Even though I had been trained to handle all these vehicles, I would find any excuse to trade routes and buses because I was terrified of the Cherry Avenue stoplight. I was terrified of getting stopped at the top of the hill with other vehicles behind me. What if I can't pull off from the stopped position? What if I panic and stall? Rather than finding out the answers, I rather trade routes. My supervisor got hip to my actions and issued a strong warning "if you try to trade again you will be terminated." Joe and I have been friends for a while, we met when I started attending PVCC years ago at night and he drove transit route #7. The following Monday I was assigned a route that had a permanent bus, the Prospect Avenue route which was riddled with stops on or near hills. The bus was an automatic bus 740. Two days after taking over from the regular driver the bus broke down and I was forced to drive 704 a stick shift. I had come face to face with my nightmare. No time to get scared if the bus broke down I had over 20 children on board. Nothing like being forced to confront your fears head on, I had to keep reminding myself that I would've been denied my CDL (commercial driver's license) if I was unqualified. Mr. Stratton, the training supervisor had more confidence in my skills than I. By the end of my middle school run I had gotten a little more comfortable but the test was still coming, my high school route had stops on hills and to travel the twist and turns of Rio Road. When I returned to the bus yard a few of my coworkers cheered, laughed and teased me. Joe pulled me aside and asked how it went. My reply was "I didn't run over anyone today, yet."

When the challenge was first proposed I was still bumming rides, riding public transportation and seeing Emmett who gave me rides to work, school and even took me home for my birthday. Before him, I was happy catching the street and Greyhound buses anywhere and everywhere. The night that it all started to unravel began with a blow up over the usual stressors, the last minute hairdos and baby mama drama. All the day before was spent in the laundromat doing laundry for eight people. Someone else was supposed to do the oldest two girls' hair but their father didn't come up with the money to pay for the appointment. They wanted to have their hair professionally cut and permed for school pictures. To have their plans doused abruptly made them want to lash out against authorities. Usually I'd try to play peacekeeper but I was determined not to intervene. Having to humble themselves and ask me to help angered everyone. Tempers flaring made me clean house or attempt to. I told everyone to leave and take everything they owned. I had grown tired of being the only adult in the relationship, or at least that was how I was feeling. Maybe I should have planned a little bit before leaving myself ride-less on Monday morning. Nonetheless I slept good Sunday night. Early Monday morning I called in for the morning shift but Joe sent someone to pick me up and arranged for Mr. Willis to take the boys to daycare. Starting Tuesday I had to leave home by 6:25 which took a great effort only because every day to get to work on time me would have to catch a ride with a coworker. In order for this miracle to happen daily I would get up at five, shower, dress, pack lunch and wake the boys. Getting two sleepy children dressed and expecting a three year old to walk fast enough to catch Mr. "nothing but on time" Green to work had to be a miracle. Lugging a car seat, pushing a stroller and begging Demetrice to hurry up rounded my before 6:30 a.m. routine Monday through Friday.

Every day for about two weeks I have passed a house with a Toyota Celica in the yard for sale and I never really paid attention until now. Nothing like necessity to make a person open their eyes. I stopped to find out the price at 8:50a.m and returned with the $250 before 10a.m. I hurried to the DMV and by 1:30 I was experiencing something brand new to me, total freedom. Freedom, independence, ownership not only of a car but of my life and time. The freedom to go and come as I wanted without the restrictions of time and worrying about someone else's vehicle in my possession. When Emmett came to pick me up with an already crowded car it felt good to dismiss him. I picked up the kids from daycare with a different mentality and attitude that afternoon. Usually as soon as I hit the door of the Teal room the race against the clock was on. I had just under 20 minutes to collect the children from two different classrooms, be packed and ready to travel 4 blocks or more to the bus stop in order to catch the correct transfer route so not to be stranded for an hour and a half because the bus that came the closest to my house only ran on the odd hours. Or I had to hurry because I was on someone else's schedule. To finally have time enough to actually chat with their teachers and administrative staff because again I was looking for a part- time job felt so good, even liberating. Something to do during the middle of the day after the morning school bus runs from 9:30-1:30, odd hours to try to fill without having to promise to return to complete some 8 hour shift somewhere. At first it was slow going to pick up any hours so I volunteered and when the teachers realized I was artistic everyone wanted me to sub, hoping I would create something magical on their classroom's bulletin board. After a while the administrative staff had me coming in every day regularly during that 4 hours and also from 4:30 until 6, which was perfect. It gave me 9 ½ hours daily Monday through Friday; a 40+ hour work week with weekends off. Thankfully it also turned into my snow day and summer job because at the end of the school year my school bus job ends. Since I'm still one of the newest drivers on the team, I'm only assured a returning position for fall, not for summer school. I thank GOD because he always provides what you need, maybe not the moment you ask but by the moment you really need it.

What the difference a day can make. I hadn't had my licenses for six months before getting a ticket. I always secured my children into their safety seats and usually know my speed, this day both came into play. Traveling away from Grady Avenue store one evening after picking up the kids something to snack on during the 2 hour ride to Emporia a policeman pulled me over and swore that I was going 35 in a 15 zone and also Demetrice had taken his seatbelt apart looking back at the officer after we were stopped and that got another charge tacked on before he finished writing the ticket. Even though I protested because he was wearing it until we were stopped. I think he saw an opportunity to fill that quota even though no policeman will admit they have a quota or that they're especially hard on commercial drivers. So disappointed about the ticket I canceled my travel plans. By Sunday I found out that the ticket was a blessing in disguise. On my way to church going down 64 towards Louisa my car started to lose power, fortunately I was able to get off the highway and take back roads and route 250 whose speed was slower. If I had gone home on Friday it's no telling what stretch of highway my car may have totally died on. After church the car seemed okay to drive back home. I'm so thankful for the course of events that spared us some kind of accident. Although no one should ever expect a used car to perform as well as a new one would I was new to ownership. I realized quickly that a get around town car was what I owned and I had to look for another one soon. I hit the classified ads and found a '78 mustang another $250 get around for the time being. I realized that any family situation with more than one child needed three vehicles at least. Quickly after Emmett's car stopped running I found out what an imposition it was to share one vehicle. Still enjoying my new found freedom, the few minutes alone time between point A and point B a day. I felt the encroachment and became hostile. I guess that even though we navigated these waters carefully I began remembering the pull in so many directions by my own family obligations, work responsibilities, trying to maintain our love life and his children. I was trying hard not to become overwhelmed again. Because I'm notorious for piling too much onto my proverbial plate. I don't mind it when the pressure is from potential money making opportunities. So attempting to avoid any taxing I quickly picked up a second beat-around until I filed taxes. Still afraid of on the road desertion I rented cars to travel to Emporia for over a year and getting tired of putting up a $500 deposit for a weekend visit home every month I finally broke down and started looking on February 2, 1992. March 10th I test drove 3 different cars before finding my little puddle jumper, a Mazda GLC hatchback. The cutest little light blue 5-speed yes a 5-speed car. The shifting of gears has become easier and I'm addicted. In my case a shifting kind of car keeps me busy enough while driving so that I don't get bored. Yes it was a used car but it was from a reputable car dealer with a warranty and payments. Finally a reliable car that I can trust on the highway.

Why is it that you never grow up enough for your parents to quit worrying about you? One weekend when I went home my mother called the police on me. As I've always done since becoming old enough to work I had over extended my work week. Working every waking hour it seemed. Instead of making those deadbeat dads pay more child support I had taken another part time job working at Martha Jefferson Hospital in the transportation, nursing and cuddle care departments. I had been working around the clock for three weeks and promising mom I would come home for over 3 months. I swore that as soon as Demetrice stepped off the school bus I would be leaving to come home. Of course being dog tired I fell asleep and didn't leave until 6:30. I called the moment I was ready to leave, hoping to ease her worrying mindset to no avail. Almost to the turnoff of Emporia I passed a van broken down on the side of the road and about a half mile later passed a mother and two small children walking towards the exit. Immediately I pictured myself being her. I couldn't continue on without going back to see if I could help, so I turned around and went back past her on the opposite side. Turned around again to catch up to her. Just as I would be she was hesitant to get into the car without me getting out and explaining. It was already dark, cold, and starting to rain. So after soothing her fearful mind we're off to the service station. This was a time before cell phones. On the way to the service station I found out that she was headed just outside Emporia but ran out of gas with no gas can or money. To me it was a "no brainer" get her enough gas so she could get her family safely home, I would hope had it been me someone would have done the same for us. I purchased 3 gallons of gas in an old antifreeze jug and treated all six of us to a hotdog and then we all piled back into my puddle jumper to trek back to her vehicle. Once back at her car we had to MacGyver this gasoline into her weirdly positioned gas tank. After a few minutes of struggling and praying that the gas would be all she needed to get back underway, her van cranked and I followed her back to the filling station and put another five more dollars of gas in her tank. By this time it was almost 10:00p.m. By now my mother could only imagine I was dead somewhere along the way and had enlisted the help of the state police to find my missing lifeless body and kidnapped children. As I returned to my car I was met by Officer Matt Roundtree asking for identification and after verifying that I was who I said I was, he gave me 1 piece of advice "call your mother." I went back inside and telephoned before leaving. I can understand why she could be so worried after all the school bus dropped the children off at 2:30 and she knew I wasn't driving the school bus in Charlottesville that day. So in her perfect world I should have gotten on the road by three and pulling into her yard by 6. Bus drivers have to be very time aware to get children to three different schools that begin within 30 minutes of each other. I was a punctual creature Monday through Friday but when I clock out at 4:00 no more worrying until Sunday morning when I do the church transportation. Sometimes during my free time I don't even wear my watch.

    The weekend proved to be challenging because we spent the better part of Saturday evening in the emergency room with Dameon's asthma flaring up. Usually keeping him and Grey ghost (the cat) in separate rooms he could get through the weekend. With every season change it seems to become worse. Although usually contained and controlled by albuterol inhaler and rest, he has struggled to get well. Dameon struggling to breathe takes a lot out of the whole family. Demetrice has been a trooper putting up with his brother's baby reemergence. When he was an infant trying to fall asleep he would suck his left thumb and play with the ear of whoever was holding him or his brother's ears if he would come close enough. Most nights it would be his brother's ear while enjoying a bedtime story. Only on the worst nights did he play with my ears because the three of us would be in the bathroom with the shower steaming. Dameon and I would sit on the side of the tub and Demetrice would sit on the floor beneath the sink. You feel the most helpless when one of your children is struggling to catch their breath. His pediatrician was encouraging when he assured me Dameon would grow out of it.

The weekend never lasts long enough. I've always gone home on Friday evening and had to leave early on Sunday. By the time I get to my oldest son's grandmother's house and spend an hour or more trying to convince him to come to grandma Walker's house with us it's already bedtime. Spending another hour talking to mom and tucking the boys in I'm really ready to drop also. Anyone who thinks driving is an easy job is sadly mistaken. Sitting in the same position for hours concentrating on the next stretch of road. Paying attention to the crazy driver that keeps tailgating and little old people with cars so large that you struggle to see their short stature inside looking through the steering wheel going 15 miles slower than the posted speed limit in the fast lane.

With each pick-up or drop-off on the school bus or the church bus you worry about your passengers crossing the street. I now truly understand why mom didn't even want to go to the store in the evening during the week.

Upon my mother's request I agreed to start coming home twice a month. Neither one of us could have predicted the backlash this would cause. Because in order to work only every other weekend I'd have to leave one of my part time jobs. If I cut hours I work, the fathers were going to need to pay their fair share and this news was met with opposition from both dads. First Charles begged for an out of court agreement, which I accepted because he at least did make the already ordered amount and pick Demetrice up on most weekends. I knew if need be I could at any time request a review and receive a favorable judgment with arrearages because of his job change over a year prior. I knew JC was not going to be as willing so after asking and receiving one of his usually flippant answers, I filed for more benefits because the voluntary method hasn't worked yet. Why is it that when asked for more money, absentee parents think they can provide better care, than the primary? As if to do what they should already be doing is a huge request for an internal organ. Because of the request for more child support, we're in and out of court it seemed every month.

Thinking that he would make me angry he requested visitation. The judge granted him every other week custody, with me retaining physical custody. That meant that every week we would exchange custody at the daycare center. The daycare center was the constant in Dameon's life according to the judge. In the event that he was going to be absent, the parent that had him that week had to call the other parent and also notify the daycare center. Each week on Friday evening the other parent would pick him up from the daycare. I knew that this was going to be a bad situation, but you can't go against the judge's wishes. Dameon would be fine and have an uneventful week when he was at home with me. Unfortunately the same did not prove to be the truth in his father's care. It seemed that every week he either came home with a cold or a new bruise. After documenting incident after incident, I grew more and more angered with Judge Janine Shannon. I tried several times to petition for a protective order, decision reversal and not to have to send Dameon back to his father's house. But of course something drastic had to happen before she would listen. The story I was given was that he struck paper matches, set the trash can on fire and then sat down on the trashcan. All of these actions take precision for an adult, so imagine that the above actions are being done by a 21 month old baby. So ask yourself, does this make sense? The message I received down played the severity of his injuries. By the grace of GOD Dr. Benjamin was the pediatrician on duty when he was taken to the doctor. He was the go to doctor about child abuse for Martha Jefferson Hospital. When he saw Dameon that Tuesday morning he dressed the wounds and demanded to see him again on Wednesday morning. I was having no luck in reaching his father for answers so I called the doctor's office and pretended to have forgotten the time to bring him back on Wednesday. That was the longest twenty hours of my life. I took the morning off from the school bus thinking and praying JC wasn't lying when he said in that nonchalant message that Dameon had a minor accident with some matches. Who would've thought when I woke up that Wednesday morning that by 10 o'clock I would be on house arrest at University of Virginia Hospital emergency room for threatening the lives of three people? Anyone in my position would've been as outraged as I was. When Dr. Benjamin unwrapped the bandages he could tell that something more than just a simple burn was going on. Upon discovery he told me to take Dameon directly to UVA that they would be expecting him. While I scooped my child and his belongings, his stepmother continuously declared she would never do anything to harm him, Judas.

Upon arriving at the totally packed emergency room when I told the registration lady his name we were surrounded by nurses and the police. We were taken into an exam room that had lots of lights set up shining straight at the stretcher. Once in the room the attitudes and atmosphere changed. A nurse stripped my child from my arms and one of the officers grabbed me. Within five minutes they had taken pictures that revealed two things: first that his burns were third degree burns and also that he had been beaten with a leather strap after being burned. This angered me so that I threatened to kill his father, stepmother and that crazy judge. Immediately Dameon was admitted to the Decamp burn unit. I was placed on house arrest in the hospital room and given stern instructions not to leave the building, as if I was going to let my son out of my sight, again. He got spoiled by everyone because he was the youngest patient they had ever taken care of. While hospitalized Dameon had an IV hindering the use of his right hand which forced him to develop his left, still to this day he writes as a leftie. After a lengthy stay in the burn unit Dameon was discharged home with me and his father's privileges were stripped until Dameon was old enough to choose for himself whether to associate with that side of his family. While dealing with Dameon's hospitalization and my house arrest I had plenty time to ponder my direction. I decided to make my employment with the daycare and MJH my primary sources of income at the end of the school year. This decision allowed me to be close enough to where the boys were to maintain my sanity, them to feel secure and far enough away not to stifle or hover. After about six months of bandages and creams Dameon's scars have almost all lost their scabs revealing healthy pink, beige or brown slightly puffy cells, I remember being in awe of this. Each new day, week and month that passed I was able to step further into the shadows and watch all my children spread their wings and become stronger, more confident, independent individuals. This was comforting and concerning as well, I was about to be replaced as the most important or influential force in their lives.

By the time school resumed things were getting back on track, Demetrice was starting kindergarten and Dameon was in the blue room with Miss Deborah, a lady from my church, someone I trusted would carry out my wishes. I also found another parent and grandparents to trade off with. I would drop the boys off in the morning with the grandparents of a classmate of the boys. Demetrice would catch the school bus with the older sister and Dameon and the younger sister were taken to daycare by the aunt and most evenings I would pick up the youngest from daycare and exchange her at the older children's after school program. This worked so well, I rem

I started going to bingo just as an outlet, with a coworker. Who knew that I'd catch the bug? I guess anyone that played bingo ever would tell you your first solo win will be the one that gets you hooked. It's the building anticipation, the adrenaline rush, and the sweet release of yelling BINGO! I would imagine some could compare bingo to sex: anticipation, climax and relief or further frustration of waiting for one number as some person across the room screams BINGO! I was trying to defeat the boredom of the weekends without the kids when things were good. During that time the occasional win made the time away fun. I found myself wanting to go more frequently, the twice a month on Saturday evening turned into every Saturday. I also went sometimes on Friday nights, not so bad right? Just like any addiction once in a while became a five day a week habit. I had found myself a new source of income as well as fun. There's somewhere to play bingo every day of the week, even Sunday.

My mom was a queen of many things, most of all deception. The weekend that I realized she no longer drove the school bus I was led to believe that she retired because she was tired of doing the very job she once called the best job second only to being a mother. Inside I'm sure in my heart I knew she was perpetuating a fraud. She volunteered to keep the boys for a week; to further sell this lie. I hadn't been home for a day before someone was ready to leave. Tuesday after work Debbie, a coworker at the daycare rode with me to pick them up. A run down and back took 5 hours. Mom got mad at me for not forcing the boys to stay. Why is there a double standard implied and expected for grandmothers? It's like all the rules got rewritten, and the guilt trip that gets thrown. I was very smart for taking Debbie with me because mom would have persuaded me to stay overnight and leave early in the morning. So many times over the years my mom and I left conversations unfinished, this was one of those times. Looking back I think this was a test for her to figure out two things; whether Dameon's asthma was going to tolerate Grey ghost and whether she would be able to tolerate the boys around permanently. I know now that she had started to take stock of her life but realizing Dameon's asthma wasn't going to survive the cat long. She chose not to tell me how serious her health problems were. I wish so many days over and over that she would have trusted me with the truth. Had I been trusted with the realistic happenings I would like to think that I would have had the intestinal fortitude to pick up my life and go home to try to be some sort of help to mom, had she allowed. What I later came to find out was that she had her first heart attack behind the wheel of the school bus in 1992. Having this new information scared me into trying to be more available for mom. Every second and fourth weekend I would go home to help mom or just to ease my mind.

The winter of '93 was especially harsh but my little puddle jumper never got stuck though. For much of that time we spent 24/7 at Martha Jefferson Hospital because the weather kept school closed for almost two weeks. I needed an income and because Dameon's asthma was at its worst. Thankfully MJH cared about their loyal employees and really understood how important family was. 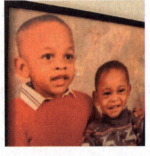 While Dameon was hospitalized Demetrice was allowed to camp out with him, which allowed me to continue to work my regular schedule and even as much overtime as I wanted. I finally embraced adulthood in that period—something about being able to pay my bills with one paycheck made me comfortable. Tired of paying for minor repairs on my trusty puddle jumper and thinking things were good, I broke down and went looking for a Jetta. I had seen the new models and fell in love. NOT really wanting to assume a car payment over $200 I continued looking for a few months. After being told that I needed a front axle and it would be over $1500 to replace; I hastened my search. My father used to say once minor repairs turn into major it's becoming a money pit. Still wanting a Jetta I continued looking at every dealership in Charlottesville until deciding my budget wasn't Jetta worthy because I didn't want to need a second income to ride in style. Finally I found a 92 Mazda at Brady-Bushy Ford. Although not a Jetta; it had everything I set out looking for. It wasn't showroom brand new or current year but it still had pristine interior and low mileage. It also was a four door money green 5 speed Protégé with much needed arm and leg room. The price tag said $13,500+ and the salesman was saying the right things. It was parked in my parking space by 5:30. I called my girlfriend Etta W. about bingo that evening just as I've done every Thursday for over a year, never did any wonky meter or any real significant signs of jealousy pop into my mind but we all know how bad my intuition was at that time in my life. By the following Thursday she had succeeded in buying a newer car and tainted her husband's already suspicious mind against me further. I never understood his mentality but maybe I intimidated him because I wasn't married or maybe he had just cause because every time my then boyfriend stranded me somewhere by stealing my car I would call her to pick me up from wherever I was and being a good friend she would justify it by saying she's bail us out before and she's got them boys. I'm not sure but I suspected that my name was tied to more disappearances than just emergency pickups or bingo evenings. No assuming PLEASE! I don't think she was cheating – I just think that my new found freedom reminded both of them of days gone by and amplified their individual fears. Her fear of loss youth and freedom. Along with homemaking, 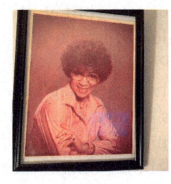 mothering and being a wife she had to trade her free days for full time employment; the very things that made me feel complete and sane made her frustrated and crazy. He saw inadequacies in himself after a car accident on his way to work one night which totaled the family vehicle and all the progress they'd made in rebuilding after financial setbacks; he didn't care about keeping up with the Jones he just wanted to never be evicted or have to borrow from me again.

By February 1994 mom had quit working totally because her health had deteriorated to the point of needing dialysis three days a week. I was driving the school bus that Friday morning when my boss radioed for my location and sent someone to relieve me. The whole drive back to the school bus yard my heart pounded as if it was coming out of my chest. I couldn't imagine what was wrong, only knew that there was trouble somewhere. JoeJoe met me outside and gave me the news that my mom had been admitted to Nash General Hospital in Durham North Carolina because of a heart attack. She got lucky because she was in her doctor's office when it happened. So, I went and rented a car because mine was having work done. Usually I'd rely on reports from my aunt or cousin during the week but this time my mother was trying to check out of the hospital AMA (against medical advice). When she makes up her mind about something there's no changing it. I was the only one that could talk some sense into her. In my haste to get home I was passing everything on the highway until I blew past a police car in Prince William County. All the information and events of the day caught up with me at that moment, when he pulled me over I broke down in tears and couldn't formulate enough words to say my mother had a heart attack and I'm trying to get there or anything. All I could do was cry. He ticketed me and said slow it down. I took the ticket and went on my way still crying hard, it had finally registered that the dynamo I call mom was human with human flaws, was slowly getting sicker, weaker and frail. For months I went home every weekend faithfully until mom got tired of us being around because it made her realize that she was sickly. She despised feeling needy but realized her level of independence was declining.

Apparently no matter how much time one has to prepare for the death of a parent it's never enough. The Tuesday morning that my aunt Buck called to tell me my mom had passed, it hit me like an anvil. I had just left from seeing her on Sunday, she was back in the hospital again but it had gotten easier to deal with because she had snapped back so many times before. Looking back now I realized she was trying to ready me for just this day because she kept telling me information that I would need after her death and telling me she was tired. Also she asked for some bananas I knew no better back then, but as I said things were done on Barbara's terms and time. I didn't know that she had signed a DNR (do not resuscitate) order, she knew I would not want that but it wasn't up to me. Quickly I had to adjust my feelings and accept that she knew that she didn't want to go on in the condition she was in. She was supposed to come home on Monday but instead of having to return on Tuesday for dialysis the hospital decided to keep her until after the treatment, she passed during dialysis.

No sooner than she took her last breath, the vultures of the family began picking through the little belongings she still possessed as though the crown jewels were hidden on that property. Back on April 26, 1995 having just buried my mother and childhood pet both on that day, I realized I no longer had a place to call home. I closed the door on my childhood and embraced adulthood officially because from that moment on it was just GOD, my children and me because the rest of my mother's distant family wasted no time letting me know I didn't belong. The one unfortunate thing was my mother had predicted this the week prior to her death and she did her best to prepare me.

April 27th quickly showed me that life doesn't care what happened yesterday it just went on, that Friday started with uncovering a snake's nest in the old house while trying to retrieve some items I wanted from my childhood. The past sometimes is best left buried in the past because the way you remember and preserve it may be different than the way it's recorded or remembered by others. Luckily I looked before reaching. I also realized that anything and everything would bring me to tears and most days did. I had lost so many things in that last week. My mother and I may have bumped heads on some things but she was more than just mom; she was a friend, an inspiration, my greatest cheerleader and my rock. After dad had been gone a few months the climate changed between us. I think we both did some maturing because we recognized the glue that bound us as a family was no longer there and we we're alone. Although we were strong individuals, we knew there's more strength in numbers. Unfortunately losing her made me lose my way to the point that I couldn't trust those around me. I was so broken that I didn't even trust my own intuition. This set me up to be robbed by the person in my bed, and made me wonder if I was being paranoid. I didn't want to accuse, be wrong and drive him away because I had a real fear of being alone. Even though I was in this relationship with someone I'd known for years I was unequally matched. Although we're only two years apart in age we were years apart in maturity. Most of the time his antics could be overlooked but with my nerves frayed and my mind fragile anything that usually made me laugh now just made me cry, angry, or lash out. Not realizing depression as such I was allowing more than I usually would withstand.

    At the time of my mom's death I was already running on fumes because of an oversight on my part. I totally forgot about the court date for the ticket. I only found out this by being pulled over by a Charlottesville policeman on East High Street two days after that court date. Usually things of this sort would not rattle me but I had no fight left in me. So I quietly accepted my fate and paid the ticket and went on with my life or so I thought. Had I'd known that the ticket possessed the power to wreck my whole earning potential as I knew it at that time I might have found the strength to protest. You see the ticket was for speeding of course but what I was unaware of was anything over 80 mph on the interstate is considered reckless driving, that cost me two of my jobs. Because I didn't show up to court my license was suspended thereby leaving my boss at the school bus job no room to defend my employment after a minor accident. I also lost the driving position with my church, which hurt but I understood both job's position because of insurance and liability, I was entrusted to transport people from five to seniors and nobody wants to receive news that there was an incident that caused injury to a loved one especially if the operator wasn't legally licensed.

    Feeling trapped in a never ending nightmare and becoming nauseated every night when I walked through the doors of Martha Jefferson Hospital to do a job that just six weeks prior I truly loved, but now can't find interest or peace. I would clock watch and every conversation that used to bring smiles now seemed to be forced. I realized that being in healthcare wasn't rewarding, interesting or even fun right then and it became apparent to my supervisors as well. My work performance has become difficult to handle because I don't sleep well when off and sometimes I would sneak off to the transportation office and take a nap during my lunch break. I began asking the floors to page me if they needed my help before I arrived. Then eventually I found it so hard to enter the ICU department without crying, I had to avoid contact and conversations which was almost impossible because a secretary needs to be polite, helpful, reachable and punctual; I had become the exact opposite withdrawn, unreachable, and tardy. Often by the time I visited the floor the nurses had completed most of the paperwork needed. I was aware that I should have been more available to them but my mother's plight weighed heavily on my mind always and if a patient was dying I just cried the whole time I had to be on that floor. Eventually it got so bad I started calling in saying I was sick. I still wasn't thinking depression had taken over my life because I was too knowledgeable to sink there again, right? Truth is the depressed person is the last one to know. Depression slowly takes over like alcoholism, starting with one simple symptom: not enjoying talking and not being able to function without crying over the time span of six weeks it grew worse daily.

Chapter 4: The beginning of the Latter

Again I need to reinvent the wheel, myself, and the family budget. With lack of definite direction I applied at Adams & Garth temporary service, I figured with my laundry list of experience that I would not have trouble finding work. I immediately got assignments that were a day here and there that covered small things but this worried me because I'm used to knowing where my rent money will come from. The last Wednesday in that month I found myself sitting in the middle of my bed with a stack of bills and only a $35 child support check to pay them. I did the only thing I knew to do in that situation, in my left hand the check and in my right the bills I lifted them high and asked GOD to turn that money into enough to cover those bills. I said if he would I would faithfully tithe and tell everyone about this blessing from that day forward. My friends, GOD showed up and showed out; I took that $35 to bingo and GOD turned it into over $800 for the bills, tithes, and enough to play bingo again the next night this went on for over 3 years. The Lord also blessed me with continuous work through the temp service until my head was back straight and the depression had subsided. I was fortunate enough to work at ConAgra through the temp service for more than a year until five days before they closed their doors for good, even after other temps had been let go. From there on Friday to a new assignment at Figgie on Monday that lasted until December 1997. All in all, the Almighty has always provided everything I've ever needed!

On January 5, 1998 I began working at Craig Builders as a receptionist. This job was right for me in many ways. It offered: the perfect hours, no more babysitter or afterschool unless I wanted. I got to wear heels and dresses instead of hairnets, earplugs, steel toe shoes and the safety goggles of the last two jobs. Also I was doing something that I enjoyed. I was being trained to do accounts payable accounting. AP accounting is more than just writing a check to a supplier or to a construction worker because everything has to be accounted for on every invoice and expense sheet. Although one roofing nail may only cost a fraction of a penny, imagine how many go into building just one house and at any time there were at least four houses being renovated or built. Each piece of material had to be counted even down to each pound of nails. So used to working 8 or 12 hours a day, on March 17th I went back to the office after scooping the boys from school to chat with my immediate supervisor and the owners about taking on more responsibilities and my 90 day evaluation, which for probably the first time ever I was confident. Little did I know how drastically different my life would become in less than eight hours.

I've never been good at clean breaks even when the writing was on the wall in neon! The guy that I had been seeing for three years was two and a half years past his usefulness. I adored his mother and the rest of his family. Maybe still missing my own mother I found a suitable substitute with great family values but different enough to not ever replace or make me feel guilty. I know that I stayed in that shamble of a relationship because of two things: her and the love of fishing. We seem to live on some river bank every weekend. The James, the Hardware, Lake Anna, the Reservoir or Reyes Fjords, if it had fish we were there all year round. My children seem to enjoy it so despite my initial protest I finally got on board.

The day of my accident started as many before, I didn't have my own car once again. I hoped on Sunday that Sterling was going to manage to keep his word and just go exactly to point B and back, yet again he failed. In past incidents I've gotten left at work, being forced to catch the bus, left at his mother's house forced to stay overnight and lied to about these actions. It's now Tuesday, without even a call on Monday even though it would have been a lie. Had the reason been another woman I would've had no problems walking away but ...I'm a fixer, a warrior, a worrier and a fool. I used to believe that with love, prayers, and support that he could and would beat his addiction, little did I know that trying to be understanding and supportive was blocking blessings. Thinking a few months back that if he had his own car again it would eliminate my problem, well most of the time it did. This was one of those between times; you know one of those times that everything seemed fine for a week or more and then out of nowhere you get hit by a curveball, blindsided, hoodwinked or just thrown for a loop. Faith and love for his family made me keep grasping at that glimmer of hope just to be let down again. When finally you've reached your limit and realized that there was no change going to happen unless you made the change occur. So to gather my thoughts before breaking the news I decided to go to the one place that helped me think things over other than prayers, bingo. Being the way I was led to my downfall. Instead of pulling up my big girl panties when he strolled in so unconcerned that he had yet again broke his promise to his mother and my heart, I couldn't find the courage to just say **ENOUGH AND GET OUT!** Instead I asked him to watch the kids so I could go to bingo. Usually when I would ask the household if I could go to bingo I would meet opposition from everyone but not that time. I left home with $20, my bingo bag, licenses and bank card. I stopped by the bank intending on getting another $20. After sitting waiting for 15 minutes for my turn at the ATM I decided against withdrawing more money. Unfortunately I didn't listen to that little voice saying go home and deal with my problem. Instead I looped back around and got on 250 heading for the Moose Lodge in Keswick, never to arrive. It had begun to rain lightly, just enough that it combined with oil and gas on the road made the surface slippery. Usually I would be speeding or at least going faster but this time I was in no hurry. Although I was in the fast lane, when a police car approached flashing its lights, I changed lanes and they sped by. Unfortunately as I changed lanes my car began to hydroplane. Having driven everything from a Pinto to a school bus and everything in between I knew not to fight the water beneath my tires. I let the car drift off the right shoulder to gain traction before pulling back onto the pavement. Maybe I should have come to a complete stop before continuing on but yet again hindsight is 20/20. As I pulled back on the road I started to hydroplane towards the median and a huge dirt pile. Then I did jerk the steering wheel to try not hit the dirt pile head on. For a long period of time I used to rack my brain wondering what else if anything I could have done to avoid that accident, short of staying home.

Nonetheless I clipped the dirt pile with my front left tire as I jerked the wheel; that was enough to flip the car one full turn and a half. As the roof above my head made contact with the pavement it crushed. I remember my forehead hitting the dome light and my body feeling as you do on a loop of a roller coaster, my bottom losing contact with the seat. The thrust and the twirling was disorienting but I never lost consciousness. Even though I was alert when the car finally came to a stop I had no idea that the car was resting on the passenger's side with the driver's side in the air. As I realized the accident was over, I had the idea to sit up and assess the damage. Just then I felt a cool, calming hand touch my left cheek as though to say be still; so I did just that. I'm not sure of how long it took for someone to come to help but eventually I heard someone telling me that they had called 911 and authorities were on the way. They also called my family for me. I'm very grateful for those two good Samaritans because I had heard other vehicles going past after the accident at least twice. Everyone that rubbernecked and kept on going had to be on their way to bingo. Anyone that didn't pass that area before the EMS crew got there didn't get through for over two hours or more.

Shortly after that it was off to the races, East Rivanna Fire Company the one that holds bingo on

Monday nights and Charlottesville Albemarle Rescue Services (CARS) were hard at work with the Jaws of Life struggling to free me from my mangled and twisted tomb, I used to call my baby. Before starting to cut Me out they stabilized my non- existing neck with a pediatric collar in the front and a full-sized adult back piece. After opening up my car like a tuna can we all faced the reality of paralysis when one of the first responders asked me to push with my feet. We made eye contact and before I could say I'm trying, even among the raindrops, I saw a tear roll down his cheek. You see, although a volunteer fireman he also works for the E-911 call center of which for over three years had been the one job that has eluded me. The next day would have been my sixth interview and he was one of the people that conducted those very interviews. I was always told to keep applying because I was qualified but kept losing out to people with more experience because they held that same or similar position elsewhere. I had been pursuing this position so long and acing the entrance exam in the top 5 percentile of the country each of the three times I was tested. Therefore when the job was re-listed Naomi from Human Resources would just call me and ask if I wanted to reapply, then forward my application over to the interviewers at the E-911 call center; of which I was to interview with again on the 18th.

Forgive me I got lost on another insignificant story yet again, back to the scene, after realizing I had a neck injury EMS decided street transport was too dangerous so Pegasus was dispatched. I was informed of this determination after their initial assessment and extrication. My vital signs had been very good throughout the whole ordeal until this news. I was told that they needed to place an oxygen mask over my face because the downdraft of Pegasus's propellers would take my breath away as I was being loaded. I was alert and oriented. The approaching mask seemed to make me feel claustrophobic, which brought on a panic attack. My blood pressure shot up to 250/137. This was the first realistic look into my new life ahead but still the seriousness was a ways off yet. The trip from the crash site to the hospital helipad took less than five minutes, to be honest all of my panicking was unnecessary. I remember a slight gravitational pull on liftoff and a small landing touchdown, nothing like anticipated, but not a ride that I would want to retake. Once on the helipad a team of people grabbed the Stretcher and ran with it toward the emergency department doors. I was taken to one of the trauma rooms of which I've spent many hours in but never as the patient. I am transferred to the hospital stretcher. The trauma team kicked into high gear right away while one person started an IV line another was destroying my favorite bingo outfit: my black faded glory jeans, a red T-shirt, and my black Reebok high tops, all cut off...up one side and down the other. Because of the injuries from the accident being careful to remove the garments properly was undoubtedly not feasible. Minimal movement until X-rays and a battery of other scans could reveal all the injuries. I remember being strapped to the backboard and following sounds and movement with my eyes. What I can't remember is feeling pain, cold, or scared. For the most part I still felt calm and serene but inquisitive.

After hours of tests I was admitted to the MICU (medical intensive care unit) where I was being observed. I remember thinking they're rolling the dice to see if I'm going to make it. While they hoped the swelling would go down and things would improve. I wasn't able to move without assistance because of a "halo" with weights attached so I couldn't accidentally move the wrong way and do more damage before surgery on Friday March 20th. So in order to change positioning any at all it was a four person production. My next door neighbor Anna worked at UVA hospital at the time of my accident and called my oldest son's grandma at my request on the 18th. I can remember the day that my oldest son came to see me after my accident. It was the 19th. My ex and his brother brought my then fifteen year old to see me, so he wouldn't worry. Have you ever known something but never really received confirmation until too late? I always suspected that pride and my mother kept us from getting back together. I finally got my answer that Thursday night. After the usual small talk: hi, how are you and you okay? "He went out into the hallway and cried. "NOT just the usual thug-hard guy one tear but... that I know I screwed up and I know it's too late kind of weep session" my son finally told me in 2018. That was the first time I cried since the accident also. I don't know the exact reason for my tears but this was the first moment I had laid eyes on either one of my children. It became real to me at that moment because I finally realized I still couldn't move anything. I will confess that maybe I realized that same thing that he did at the same time. We have always had that ability to read each other's thoughts. We're the only competition in each other's love life.... hell even today! With a love like ours why did he let stories come between us? Pride.... because he believed the lies my mother was spreading and wouldn't trust that he knew me better than that. Although I think mom started out loving me as best she could but I think it wavered or teetered between postpartum depressive anger and love. It was hard to distinguish each day. Maybe she should've gotten counseling after losing Warner. As the old saying goes "hindsight is 20/20." Instead of being happy that she was about to be a grandma all those years back...a full sixteen. She chose to tell lies about my leaving. She spread the rumors that I didn't want my son and didn't want to fight the custody agreement. Even though his mom knew what I had told her the day I left him with her. I know it all hit him with that same load of bricks that fell on me then too. Because my son had asked to come to live in Charlottesville with us because of his desire to attend the University of Virginia under the George Welsh program.

Finally the day of my surgery had come, while I was laying there having my 5th and 6th vertebrae stabilized one of my children's fathers was racing to the court to be granted full custody. I had no clue what was going on outside of my hospital room. Even though he had no consideration for my situation the courts did, I was never served until I was home 6 months later.

I remember thinking I should have turned around twice before the accident but over the years I have realized that God's will was done. I was always sticking with people and situations far too long anyway. Decision making was never my strong suit. Like most women ... when we love we love hard and fall too soon. Especially if you've suffered any type of losses. We don't want to grieve or inflict pain on others. There are some low-life guys that know how to spot the wounded prey. Just how much will be accepted? Sometimes we can be our own worst enemy by allowing ourselves to be used in the pursuit of love. God said if I didn't have enough brains to remove myself he would.

I never figured out what I did or didn't do during the accident. I just decided finally not to keep beating myself up over something that I couldn't go back and change. Also I decided not to take this gift lightly because God keeps on blessing me with one more day and if I keep on doing me and not what GOD wants eventually I will run out of chances. So the biggest thing I had been procrastinating about was telling this story; but that ends now.

For about a month after surgery I remained in MICU with a feeding tube, a neck brace, and I needed to be catheterized every 4 hours to urinate, being turned every two hours and having my limbs exercised every day. This became my new normalcy. I was transferred to the step-down unit in mid –April. My care team immediately started getting me out of bed into a reclining chair, slowly working my way to sitting up at 90°. Once I was able to tolerate sitting upright, the next step was to build stamina and strengthening. Especially strengthening my neck and core. Every day during physical therapy after ROM (range of motion) my therapists would sit me up on the side of the therapy bed to work on balancing myself without support. For a good amount of time I could hold myself up but I couldn't lift my head to participate in eye to eye conversations. Then that day finally came, I seem to be in my zone I was sitting upright, holding my head up and also talking to folks around me... too good to be true... entering the therapy room Chip calls my name and as I look at him he blows toward me and I fell backwards as if I was as light as a feather; laughing.

Letter to Self:

Now you find yourself in another situation, maybe by now you've figured out that operating anything with wheels is not in your wheelhouse. What's this, your tenth accident with wheels attached? Let's look back shall we:

1. **Age 5: rammed gun car into power wheel convertible and tore up knees and forehead.**
2. **Age 8 bicycle accident with Brownie, flipped over and landed on handlebars, losing more than your pride.**

3. Age 11 crashed through a fence with Caprice, just supposed to crank it up. Required 4 stitches in hand.
4. Age 14 over corrected while in the passenger seat ran in the ditch and worse, spilled boyfriend's dime bag.
5. Age 17 scraped 3 foot long scratch on car falling off of a skateboard.
6. Age 20 backed into a dumpster trying to get away from a shooting between others.
7. Age 23 hit a guardrail on Dairy Rd after sliding down an icy ramp.
8. Age 25 hit a stop sign with a mirror on the school bus, not so bad right, but lost my job.
9. Age 28 talking to passengers and driving too fast down Monticello Mt. took a ditch rather than try a curve.
10. Age 31 the monster of all, traveling on a straight highway, not speeding, but along comes drizzling rain, a cat running for its life, and another car in a much bigger hurry than me.

Here we are 22 years, 7 months, and 27 days later. Why did it take this long for this of all letters? There's the million dollar question, to which I'm still uncertain about today. Maybe by the book's end we will discover that and more about the 3 of us: me, myself and I. One thing that each accident had in

common was the emotional fight or flight response to fear, anger, or the avoidance of one or all.

WOW!! There's the short answer, but when has something ever just been that simple?

Each department in your care team has their own agenda within your overall program. The Physical and Occupational Therapists would coordinate their schedules with the medical team. The medical team consisted of doctors, nurses and psychiatrist. The nurses made sure that I knew every pill I was taking by name, dose, the reason for that medicine and side effects. At that time I was on thirty different pills: pills to help with spasms, pills to help me sleep, pills to help with moodiness and pills to keep from getting constipated. **YOU THINK!** I thought I had met everyone on my care team but little did I know, yet again another Social worker had their fingers on my lifeline. At the beginning of May I was brought face to face with something that I would have to deal with the rest of my life advocating for myself. I was roommates with a sweet lady that had been there three days longer than me, so we were at the same stages in our programs but there was three obvious differences: 1) she was able to use her limbs walk and do for herself, 2) she had family that visited every day and 3) she was white. Sorry to say that prejudices exist everywhere even in hearts of some who are in professions that are meant to serve all. If a nurse hadn't asked me four days before my round table discussions were to take place I might not have known. The same Social worker that was bending over backward for my roommates family meeting had never even introduced herself to me, or ever spoken one word any of the 50 times she had passed my bed to assist my roommate. At first I thought I was being paranoid but to test my assumption the next few times she entered the room I made a point to attempt to get her attention. I simply spoke to her and nothing twice. At first I chalked it up to possibly she didn't hear but I know she heard the second time because she was walking toward me and made eye contact. She chose to divert her gaze and quicken her pace. When it was confirmed that she was indeed the social worker that had been assigned my case, I requested someone else, a case worker that didn't mind working with people of color. I'm not sure what happened to her but I know she never returned to our room. I was reassigned to David Rodwell, a wonderful counselor who was helping with my transfer and an instrumental force to be reckoned with.

In order to meet all requirements of my program I had to venture out of my safety zones: my room, the nurse's station and the front lobby of the University of Virginia (UVA) Hospital, so for Mother's Day, Leigh my occupational therapist made it possible for me to attend church at Mount Zion. This was the kind of home going service that everyone deserves once in a lifetime (I'm glad I was alive to witness it for myself.) Everyone was happy to see me. After service so many people hugged or kissed me that I caught a terrible cold that kept me in bed for a week. I found out the week before Memorial Day that Woodrow Wilson Rehab Center (WWRC) in Fishersville Virginia had agreed to take me straight from the hospital. I still had one more outing to do to complete my program so again I enlisted the help of Leigh to take the two younger sons to see "Godzilla" while it was still in the movie theaters. It was during this movie that I realized the great lengths that I would go to, to see my children laugh and smile. Although I knew I was risking another cold and was spasmodic because of the coolness of the theatre, it was worth it to me. This was only the second time that Demetrice and Dameon had been together since March 17th. It was so noticeable that they missed me but moreover missed each other. After their fathers came to pick them up later that evening I told them the good news, they were happy to hear this because they missed our normalcy. Dameon even declared that whatever day I came home so was he because he wanted "to be where he knew he was loved". That statement brought a smile to my heart and tears to my face. I was instantly convinced that the children would adjust to our new normal and that it was going to be different; but okay.

I cannot specifically say why WWRC decided to accept me from the hospital because they had not done so in twenty years I found out later. Whatever the reason was I'm grateful. Four days before my thirty second birthday I was sent to start my new life, I was transferred on June 1st. I quickly found out how different life was going to be because I was dropped into my bed and didn't see anyone or anything except my spider infested room for two hours. This is when I realized my arachnophobia was going to be tested daily. The light above my bed had several different kinds of spiders living or sunning themselves less than three feet from my face and I can't even lift a finger to flick away the one that is crawling on my stomach upward. I was given a call bell for appearances because I rang several times to hear "your nurse will be there shortly". Believe me when I say my faith, willpower, and resolve was tested every waking moment. I found myself sleeping less and less because I would wake up and find one crawling toward my face quite often all I could do was blow at them. Thankfully the shallow breathing I was only capable of doing was enough to confuse the advancing spiders. They would stop to figure out if proceeding was the direction of travel they wanted to continue on or if retreating was the best.

Don't mistake me I'm so appreciative of the training I received from Woodrow because they made me learn how to direct my care, plan my life, and dream beyond today and tomorrow. I have been following the teachings of Woodrow every day because I'm the one in charge of my care, destiny and life. GOD has kept and protected me for 24 years 6 days and the hours, minutes and seconds mercifully keep on accruing. Each day of rehabilitation focused on creating the "Best new me" I could be. At first it was difficult, not just because of the spiders but because I wasn't prepared. Coming straight from the hospital I had no clothing, shoes, not even sanitary napkins. I had to ask my girlfriend Jessica for sleep wear for a birthday present. Because my supposed boyfriend was never around when he needed to be, I had to send someone to Walmart to purchase things that I needed. Also the first weeks were hard because I had to rely on someone to push me in a manual wheelchair. After a few days of learning the basics and getting supplies, I started to adapt and find my stride. Total independence will never be again it was a pipedream but to do all that I could myself was the ultimate goal. Even though I had to be bathed, fed, dressed and lifted into my chair; once there with assistive devices and lots of determination I could brush my teeth and wash my face, it may take way more time than it would if someone did it for me, but staff was patient with me. It was during this time that I discovered my signature extra-long drinking straw. I'm so glad that I finally got measured for a powered wheelchair, one more step closer to some kind of independence. My power chair cost more than the car that earned this permanent seat. Each week we were expected to attend at least two seminars and participate in two activities. I enjoyed the seminars because I learned things like skin care, how to network as a quadriplegic and the various agencies that work with people with disabilities. The activities didn't always interest me but they were required to finish my program. When I found out that my activities could include having the boys visit for a week I was all over this idea. I got to plan and instruct meal preparation. I was so happy to have all three boys with me on Woodrow's campus for seven days and six nights. We got to camp out in the visitor's suite. It was just the thing we all needed, we explored the game rooms, we took walks, enjoyed spending time with each other and like most vacations the week ended way too soon.

Each day usually started off the same way with one of the attendants bringing my breakfast tray into the room and placing it on my bedside table and asking "are you ready for breakfast?" Depending on whether I had an early therapy appointment or if I just didn't want to move, would determine when I said good morning. If I was hungry and really ready to get my day underway I would say good morning at 7:30 as they entered with breakfast. Otherwise I could be wide awake and no one would even know. I have had this ability since I was young, it used to be my protective escape from a promised beating by my mother. This ability over the years have gotten me spared a few times but became a useful skill for not just me, you see unfortunately when some people have evil tendencies it doesn't matter to them when the urges occur, they will steal. There was an attendant that had been a state employee for 25+ years that was stealing from me whenever she could, but I was instrumental in bringing her spree to an end once I knew who was behind my loss. One morning I woke up just in time to see her closing the drawer where I kept my purse. Later with the help of someone else I was able to confirm that again I was short $20, I guess I should be glad that she didn't take all $50. I was relieved in one way to finally know that the person that I had helped with transactions wasn't the person that stole from me and angered also to think that someone in a position to help would steal from the patients. Because if she was taking from me then there was no telling how many more she had hit over the years. In order to accuse her of anything I had to be able to absolutely prove beyond any doubt that my accusations were true. So to do this I went to the charge nurse and the D.O.N. (Director of Nursing) with my dilemma; they agreed to give me the latitude to prove my accusations within reason. So I asked Miss X to assist me with going to the cashier's office later that same day, never acting any different towards her, as not to tip my hand. On the way to the cashier's office we chatted about random things because I knew I wanted to be absolutely right, justified, and vindicated. Also I firmly believe in these two quotes: **"Keep your friends close but your enemies closer"** and **"Don't get mad, get even"**. I made sure not to give any hint that I knew she had stolen from me earlier, as a matter of fact I acted as if the $100 we received from the cashier was the only funds in my wallet, setting the stage for the upcoming performance. When returning to the unit I announced my intention of attending my therapy session with the psychiatrist and went to his office and had the D.O.N. summoned to that meeting. At this meeting we marked every bill in my wallet, all $130 with my initials (KWW) and the date 10-6-98, which would have been my mother's 66th birthday (how ironic still protecting from the grave). So for safekeeping I kept my purse with me the rest of that day until bedtime and then returned it to the scene of the crimes, yes I said crimes because all of the day's activities was to catch her the next morning. Unfortunately most kleptomaniacs will steal from someone repeatedly and almost always the same amount. In on the setup was Lorinda the charge nurse, the D.O.N., the Psychiatrist, Campus Security and of course me. Just as the previous day I didn't respond when Miss X whispered "are you ready for breakfast" and true to form she proceeded to the purse and helped herself. As soon as she left the room I rang the bell for the charge nurse to call security and the others. Lorinda also halted Miss X and asked her to assist her in my room before she had time to get the money off of her person. I told everyone why they had been called to my room and publicly accused Miss X. Security asked her to empty her pockets and that is when I declared that the money was marked with my initials on the previous day's date in the upper left corner on the reverse side. Upon examination of the $20 bill in her pocket and the twenties in my wallet security was convinced that Miss X had stolen that money from me. I'm such a softy that by the conclusion of this encounter I was in tears because Miss X was begging me not to press charges, but because it happened on state property by a state employee the police were called in to arrest Miss X. I'm a firm believer in the fact that everyone that comes into our lives for however long or short of a season it was predestined to help mold the person we're meant to be.

    I can remember the first time I experienced "the shivers" I so wanted some ice cream. After the lunchtime duties were over one of the nice attendants accompanied me to the campus store. I had been craving a Fudge-sickle, I treated us to our favorites. It was an August day so why when a gentle breeze rustled the leaves on a nearby tree did I start shivering like it was December? After Tressa finished laughing at me she told me that it was only the first of many things that would shock my system. Even some things that I usually do daily can sometimes set off my dis-reflexive episodes. I would have to fight through sometimes and figure out the causes. It could be usually traced to one of several triggers: 1) environmental- too hot or cold. 2) Positioning- not straight enough, slouching too much. 3) Wrinkles- YES the "Princess and the Pea syndrome" is real. One day after being home for months I had a doctor's appointment for a physical. When we left home I was okay but after we left the doctor's office I began sweating when I got back in the van thinking it's because it's hot. We put the air conditioning on and proceeded to Durty Nellie's to get lunch. Only two blocks from the doctor's, by arrival I was soaking wet. In order to stop I had to go down the list of usual suspects. We repositioned, I took my medicine and after much frustration I realized my right foot wasn't comfortable... my sock had gotten pulled too tight on my toes. YES really sometimes it's just that simple, but because my sensations don't take the direct route to my brain anymore it's a guessing game.

Looking for resources, housing and people to take care of me after rehab did prove to be challenging. For one thing I was new at being "the boss", although having worked in health care most of my career, it was a little different being both patient and employer. Also I was trying to conduct business in Charlottesville from Fishersville over the phone. I posted an advertisement in Charlottesville's newspaper and tried to hold interviews at Woodrow; either the timing was wrong or the pay or both. I found over the years that for every one ad I usually found that one person that wanted to work and three that had plenty of drama.

You would think that in 1998 that there wouldn't be any more housing discrimination but it still existed in Charlottesville. I was getting happy because it seemed as though my housing dilemma was over. I was promised a handicap unit in an apartment complex near the Pantops area until I showed up to pay the deposit and sign the lease. When trying to navigate my wheelchair through the narrow doorway the property manager decided I was not the right fit for that community; so she's steadily saying that it had been rented that morning but the receptionist was looking puzzled, shaking her head in disbelief. Usually when a person discriminates against someone with disabilities it's because they don't understand the disability or are just phobic. Retailers and Landlords that discriminate against individuals with disabilities can be brought up on charges under the American Disabilities Act (ADA), sometimes a fine is assessed in cases such as a landlord not renting to someone solely because of a disability and it has to be proven to be the only reason. At that time I hadn't found my voice or enough courage to fight for an unseen apartment, although it did hurt to be turned down but back to the drawing board. I asked Anne to grab a realtor's guide as we left the office. The ride back to Fishersville was especially long probably because I felt defeated, I have never before been rejected or denied housing. Another month has rolled over and desperation is setting in, after calling Janice my housing specialist, I called Four Seasons apartments and we moved in on December 7th.

The true test started Tuesday December 8th my first full day back in civilian life outside of hospital or rehabilitation facilities. No nurses, doctors or therapists to call for assistance just me, Dameon and the missing attendant from Interim nursing company. I did the only thing I could at the time, gave Dameon permission to miss school that day, called the agency about the attendant not showing up and called my evening help to make sure she was coming in that evening. Luckily I had chosen to have an indwelling catheter placed before the boys visited me at Woodrow, another step towards independence, without it I would still need to be catheterized every 4 hours. Home under fire, finally I get through to a supervisor at Interim to find out that a home visit needed to be done before an aid could start, so at least one more day on my own. Wednesday the 9th Dameon made me a peanut butter sandwich, emptied my catheter bag and tried to get me to agree with him to missing school again, as much as I wanted not to be alone, I sent him off to school. Eight until two forty-five was the longest stretch of time to me so I found it harder and harder some days to tell if I was believing Dameon's "I don't feel good "or if I was hearing myself saying I won't be alone. The agency sent someone to open my case officially on December 10th, Pete's birthday. I was so hoping that was the end of my help problems.

    Someone from church worked for Chandler, Franklin & O'Brien the law group and they persuaded one of the lawyers to take my case. I originally met the team that was handling my case when I was still hospitalized at UVA. The accident was determined to be no fault of mine but it was doubly hard to pinpoint the true blame. After many months of trying to make a case that would put Mazda on the hot seat because of the roof crushing in such a slow rollover, it wasn't proven to sustain a lawsuit for personal injuries. They felt sorry for me and decided to adopt our family for Christmas, they made that Christmas the best one my children and I had ever had. While still at WWRC I was able to do a little shopping but the law firm provided two outfits per child, shoes, accessories, food and household goods. There were so many presents you could hardly walk into the living room from the bedroom and one entrance to the kitchen was completely blocked.

After months of struggling to have attendant coverage from the agency it all became unbearable when the attendant assigned to take care of me decided to quit and steal my brand new coat after being spoken to by the agency about being late. When I told them what she did they said if I didn't see her pick it up, they could do nothing, even though I saw her walk past my bedroom window wearing it as she left. I started proceedings to change agencies and became labeled difficult to work with by that agency because they weren't trying to lose control of my case. So because of the hassle of changing agencies, after 6 months with a new service facilitating company, I began pursuing the steps to become a consumer directed individual, I figured I could do better or at least no worse than those agencies.

The boys made friends with children in the neighborhood and the house was always full of children around dinnertime. Because I loved hearing this laughter of lots of happy children, we began living on delivered meals like pizza, Chinese and subs every weekend. I would ask to meet the parents or at least one, because I wanted them to know whose house their child was at and because I could not get up and go looking for my children I wanted to know where they were when not at home. The two boy from next door became life - long friends and when in town stop by from time to time. Unfortunately people drift away over time. Most of my associates from my previous life have long since stopped calling and visiting. It was okay back then because I was content being a hermit until an attendant named Katrina H. came into my life and refused to do my shopping for me. Not only did she refuse to take a list to the store she threatened to quit if I didn't go to Walmart for the things I needed myself. I stalled for two days until she called my bluff on Thursday, April 9th 1999, the thought of my children not having Easter baskets was enough to break my opposition; I'm so grateful for her determination. Had she not forced me out I might be still finding excuses today. After emerging from my habitat and readjustments to the outside world the children and I would catch the bus anywhere we wanted to go on Saturdays during the school year, but spring break and summertime we were all over.

Back on the hunt again for those two seemingly elusive things; that permanent place to live and another attendant to help once we move from walking distance of the people that were helping because neither one drives or has to commute further than next door. Back then Craig's list didn't exist or I knew nothing about it. Back then, just as today it wasn't hard to recruit individuals that claimed to be certified nursing assistants (CNA's) but to find good ones was the challenging task. When your insurance is government provided you can be assured that one of these will happen:

    1. You will find someone wonderful but because of the low wages they'll have to move on to provide for their family or,

    2. You will find that eager beaver straight from high school that will eventually be heading to nursing school or graduating from school and worth keeping but too expensive or,

    3. You will find the fakers, the warm body that can find 50+ things to do except their job. The paycheck chaser that leaves after second payday because they've realized welfare and food stamps pay better or,

    4. You will come across flimflam artists, the ones that have enough skills to convince you that your needs are first and foremost. But eventually medicine and money start to supplement their pay. They leave after you figure it out.

My biggest fault was trying to hold on to create, shape, mold and change everyone into the attendant I wanted them to be. This almost always ended the same way, me falling for some sob story about why they are having troubles making it to work. I being change phobic would try to help and have loaned money that wasn't returned or paid bills just to have them quit right after. Looking back now I really acknowledge the fact that GOD put certain people in your life for the season that you need them, but sometimes all that came with you aren't meant to continue on your journey; realizing when to leave them behind is part of the growth process!

Finally, finding adequate housing in Rio Hill apartments takes a load off of my mind. Now only if attaining worthy assistants could become this easy. I would like to think that by now I've wised up enough to spot the good or at least enough to weed out the bad faster; but I've shown in previous pages my learning curve seems to be a straight line. I hated placing ads in the Daily Regrets (Progress), the biggest circular in this town in the early 2000's, not worth the $100+ to run an ad from Sunday to Sunday. Every time I ran the listing I would get lots of callers but most were seeking unemployment searches, not a job. Out of 20 callers I would usually get only 3 to show up for an interview and then if they came back for training maybe 1 would show up for work. I know most would say that's how it should work, yes but most of the time I was in need of two people. Even today I'm always short of backup or relief staff. It's hard to retain anyone that you can't guarantee a certain schedule. In order to employ 3 people nobody would get enough hours to live off of 1 job, hell 2 people can't live on this job alone. Over the years GOD has provided for and protected me from being reported to authorities for inadequate coverage. Even though I'm of sound mind which helped, it didn't stop a few folks from calling social services with the intention of helping or so they thought. Had they bothered to ask me what they could do to help I would have been able to save them the trouble and me too. Nothing. It never worked the way intended by well-wishers, it just got a case opened with Adult Protective Services (APS of Albemarle County) but after 2 interviews: one with me and one with the boys; it was always determined that the accusations were unsubstantiated. Usually it managed to get our names added to some Christmas or food donations lists. So looking back I should say thank you to the well -wishers and those with ill intentions because God worked it in our favor. The well-wishers always hoped their concerns would help get me more help, more hours paid for by Medicaid or any new resources that were previously unavailable to me. The ill - intentioned folks were almost always people that had worked for me and got replaced or chose to supplement their pay by stealing medicine, clothing, the kid's toys, games or money. When and if reported they would try to fabricate some sort of infraction about my hiring or payment methods as if I controlled what the agencies offered or as if I could influence DMAS.

Ever since I came back to Charlottesville I realized that to be a contributing member of society I needed to yet again attempt school or some type of training program because for me to earn enough to be self-sustaining my barely 12th grade education

(GED), some college and holes in my resume wasn't going to be enough because now no matter how much previous work experience, equipment knowledge or on-the-job training I already possessed; the first thing potential employers see is my wheelchair. I attempted to get a job that quite frankly I was overqualified for and was promised the position on the phone; just to lose it in person. Even after explaining that DRS would make sure to provide any assistive devices I would need to do the job proficiently and with professionalism. It doesn't take much too totally destroy an already fragile ego. My last employer's promise of my job being secure terrified me because I loved that job and knew all the duties like the back of my hand; I also knew my capabilities and limitations. Being honorable people I know if I showed back up they would try to make it work but for how long. I couldn't do any paper shuffling, filling was out, assistive technology would help but the only part of my previous duties I would be able to do was answering the phones. I know the Craig brothers would have no problem creating that receptionist position because quite frankly that was my title before. Maybe it was me being afraid of tiring or maybe I didn't want to feel like a charity case. Not seeing the tremendous gift it would have been and the boost for my damaged psyche I took a step back and took into account that any job could have jeopardized my disability benefits. Nonetheless I didn't return to work. I should have at least gone to visit and thanked them for their generosity because they continued to pay me for another three months the same amount of time I had been employed.

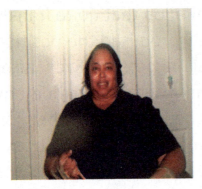

Coasting along for years living vicariously through my children, Paige Moore called me in late January 2008 and asked if I would like to participate in the Miss Wheelchair Virginia pageant at WWRC. That month flew by while I prepared. Although I had never done any type of public speaking, I decided to step out on faith, overcome my wallflower mentality for once and for all. It was a grueling weekend filled with seminars, dancing, eating and fellowship. From Friday 5p.m. to Sunday 3p.m. something to do every waking minute and I enjoyed it. Can't wait until I am able to do it again.

After that weekend my health issues began to plague me: I was diagnosed with sarcoidosis and diabetes. I have lost count of how many times I've been hospitalized because of UTI's. I have been septic to the point that I didn't know where I was or recognized my own children. In earlier infections I required a nephrostomy tube because my left kidney was blocked because of stones. Believe you me, I now know why that condition is called sepsis. You feel like you're hovering over the toilet and one more pang or twinge will just flush you away. That pain was worse than any pregnancy contraction I ever felt and never ending. I became nauseated, having chills and sweats, delirious and sometimes comatose, nothing I would wish on my worst enemy. A few of those times doctors had given up but gratefully Dr. Jesus never gave up... Thank You Lord!

Also trying to continue to eat like before I suffered with constipation. From the beginning I wasn't getting all my bowel needs met in the hospital, because I wasn't aware. I don't remember having a bowel regimen until I got to the stepdown unit but that has got to be wrong because that would mean I didn't poop for over a month. Hmmm ... I was so backed up for years *so maybe I'm not crazy*. When I wasn't getting hospitalized for a UTI it was for bowel issues. Many times after a hospitalization I would be sent home when a PICC line feeding meds directly into my heart for sometimes a month. But by the Grace of GOD I'm still here to tell the story!

Along came Julie an African exchange student that made my life so much easier, bearable and happier. She became my first live-in attendant. Mrs. U was efficient, compassionate and funny when necessary. She provided care, friendship and sisterly guidance. Mrs. U came along at the perfect time, on the heels of another string of lazy or horrendous caretakers. Most people want to work day shift, seven or eight in the morning until no later than four; anything past that hour comes with sighs, slamming doors and all out refusal. Mrs. U never complained about her duties or how long I wanted to stay up. It felt good to be able to be up to interact with the boys in the evenings until their bedtime. I loved being able to be on the computer into the late hours.

After two years and 7 months of a two bedroom apartment and many inquiries finally a three bedroom became available, now my live-in attendant can have their own room. Unfortunately, Mrs. U has finished school and returned to Africa. For 3 months I had been looking for another attendant to work evenings permanently so the new apartment allowed me to advertise differently. I ended up hiring two people but not a live-in. One of the people that I hired lived in the neighboring complex and walked to work for the first two days. The third day I got a call and she asked could her boyfriend, who I met on day 2, come because she said the lifting was too hard, so he took over her position and agreed to do 3 days and every evening shift of his days. That seemed to work for some time until the person working Monday through Thursday was injured in a car accident. Again looking for another attendant Mr. P did his very best to cover each uncovered shift because nobody lasted very long, or so I thought. Someone that had come and went got a position at HealthSouth and clued me to what Mr. P was doing. He would allow them to work a few days or even a few weeks before he would start switching days with them and telling them I requested the change; then telling me that they asked him. I found out later that Mr. P was scooping every hour possible because she was addicted to the pain pills she had been prescribed the previous year after gastric bypass surgery. Unfortunately that fact didn't surface until 3 years after meeting her, because I didn't see her on any regular basis after day two. When I called Mr. P on his activities that is why he finally disclosed this secret and how hard she was making life for him, the children and her mom. I could not exactly be mad at him for trying to provide for the family that he chose, but yet I still felt some kind of betrayal! Probably if I had reacted in kind I would have protected myself from what happened 4 months later, Miss Missy managed to steal a counter check from my bank statement. This was on the heels of me paying a $600 electric bill 3 days before Easter. Yes I hear you screaming you fool, I'll tell you how and when. First and foremost Mr. P apologized for his actions and never tampered with the scheduling again and took a part time gig with someone else to supplement his income. I agreed to help with the electric because he had not yet been paid from his other job and promised to sign over his first 3 checks as repayment, I know I know ... boneheaded! It had been a year since the last schedule incident and I had shopping to do. We sometimes went to the grocery store together during that last 3 months because his vehicle was wrecked by one of my children when the brakes failed. He covered for them so I felt some trust and loyalty was due, okay. By the time this came to light Mr. P had decided he was fed up with her behavior and promised to pay it back if I didn't send her to jail for theft. I agreed because I have a heart or because I'm soft-hearted, I didn't want to be the reason that her children got taken away from her. So to prove that he was sincere he moved in as my live-in aide, wrong he wasn't fooling me... he didn't like homelessness! Things were fine until he met his new girlfriend Miss T was a crazy jealous piece of work. She thought that the title girlfriend gave her special permission to just walk in my house without knocking and talk to me any way she desired. Somehow she fixed her mind on the notion that I was her competition, rival and enemy before ever considering the title employer. Seeing the writing on the wall, I started looking for another person to fill the soon to be vacancy. I warned Mr. P that I wasn't going to put up with her cursing me out whenever she couldn't reach him by phone. By the time he realized how crazy she was, she was well on her way of becoming baby mama number two. Crazy is as crazy does, the apple didn't fall far from the tree, yes her mother just as bad or worse because Miss T was tame when not around mommy dearest. It had become so bad that when my phone announced her number I stopped answering, unfortunately it was too late for Mr. P to adopt the same practice, although he tried. Five months into the pregnancy she convinced or just conned him into moving in with her, the brother, the mother and mom's boyfriend. The picture had definitely become clearer because she couldn't make him walk away from his job, she was going to limit his time in my presence. When he came to work at 8a.m. at 10 she would call for his lunch request. A few moments of pleasure costs him a lifetime of hassle. After I told him I wasn't going to answer her phone calls or any unknown phone numbers, she broke down and purchased a pair of cell phones. At least my phone was mine again, until their service was disconnected which seemed to happen every month. I didn't let that delude me into thinking things were going to be totally alright, I could live with having a 28 day reprieve, as long as she could control her mouth I wasn't going to be anymore bitches, sluts or motherfuckers by that poor white trash. I'm not prejudiced but I dislike rude women, I could care less about interracial couples; I hate ignorance. Things rolled on until December 2009 when the weatherman predicted a heavy snowstorm, knowing that I needed a caregiver to be able to help me, Mr. P decided to sleep over against her protest and threats. I'm grateful for his commitment or his need for a break from her. It ended up snowing everyone in for 2 weeks, when he finally dug out it was December 23rd, his and Demetrice's birthdays. When he left to cash his paycheck she never allowed him to return until January 10th by this time I had replaced him with two older women with no drama.

During that 2 weeks period I was suffering from back pain one day so I got the heating pad put on my back once I was in my wheelchair, I asked Mr. P to remove it in 30 minutes but I fell asleep and he just let me sleep, needless to say I ended up with a burn in the small of my back. I wasn't aware that I had been burnt until Christmas Eve that landed in the E.R. for a mysterious looking and smelling spot above my butt on my back that my children noticed while repositioning me 4 days later. That was the first of a few hospitalizations for a major decubitus ulcer. I was hospitalized from December 26th until January 3rd receiving antibiotics and having the hole in my back packed with a miracle cream and gauze. That treatment healed a tennis ball size sore in less time than it takes to have a baby be born full term.

When I got home I was starting over January 3, 2010 I finally got to start calling people back that had responded to the advertisement I had done before going to the hospital, which worked out perfectly because it allowed enough time lapse between placing and returning calls to dismiss the unemployment check chasing folks that only apply for the search credit. The two ladies I ended up hiring had just begun looking after resting for a month on the heels of losing their previous client. It seemed as though GOD had taken pity on me and sent the kind of help I had been praying for. I believe that HE was extra generous to me because of all I have been through and knowing my future still held many hurdles to conquer a rest period was needed to endure what lay ahead.

These women were a breath of fresh air. Altogether different from anyone else that has ever assisted me, quiet, mature, professional, proficient and Christian. The only fault I found with both of them they were too damn quiet and sensitive. They challenged my inner being in a good way, I really had to put a stop sign between my mind and my mouth, something a previous supervisor used to have to tell me way too often. Miss D would often need reassurance that she was doing a good job. She was the most fragile of the pair, never married, no children and no life. Eventually she opened up and started talking to me. After 18 months she left to care for her maternal aunt and uncle. Or that was the reason she gave me, I later heard from Miss P that she said I yelled at her. If that had been the truth why bring a birthday present after you no longer work for that person, hmmm? I think that it was 1 of the usual reasons:

1. The money wasn't stretching far enough, in previous conversations she had questions about raises and overtime or.

2. The responsibilities, my attendants have to do everything for me except chew my food. Thankfully I can still do that, or.

3. The duties were becoming too difficult, each day seemed to bring a new ailment. There's only 7 days in a week and she only had to survive 3 of them, Monday – Wednesday and every fifth weekend which would be Friday – Sunday. At least this time I recognized the writing on the wall and got in front of it. By the time she found out about whether she was going to get the position of caring for her Aunt, her replacement was already hired.

On the other hand, the other lady was probably all together as different as night and day. Miss Peaches is the most kind - hearted, compassionate, quiet (too darn quiet) woman I've ever met. I often tell her to get out of my head. Have you ever known someone that seems to know your thoughts before you do? Maybe I'm predictable, maybe too much of a creature of habit or maybe because we have been together for 8 years, whatever the reason it's comforting and

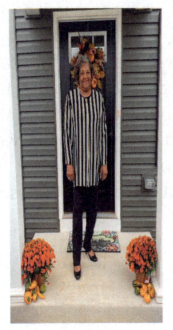

scary. She knows me better than any guy I ever dated and probably better than my children. Nonetheless I am surely appreciative of her professionalism, caring demeanor and dedication. Over these last 8 years there's never been a day that I went without coverage even when her relief didn't show. Starting July 2011 my need to hire often returned but Miss Peaches never let me worry. There's been times that Miss Peaches got off on Thursday evenings just to have to return Friday mornings. After so many call-outs and no shows, she decided to move into my third bedroom. I must admit I have gotten spoiled and relaxed having her around. I can't say thank you enough to Miss Peaches or Praise GOD enough for sending her to help. She's the kind of person that anticipates my every thought, wants and needs. This compassion and loyalty is rare in family dynamics let alone employee employer situations. As I have mentioned before I have to rely on others to be my hands which in the past has proven not to be to my advantage always, never the case with Miss Peaches if anything, I had to convince her that I trusted her. In the beginning of our relationship in order to get my bills paid she'd sit right beside me and show me every bill and check written, make a grocery list and call about any deviations. As time went on she finally settled into the knowledge that I trusted her judgment. No one will understand how freeing it is to not have to worry about the hand in your wallet, especially when you can't smack away strays. Having to depend on others to do each and every task, even simple things like brushing away a stray hair from my face, swatting a fly and opening the door to enter or exit a room or store. Miss Peaches has become someone I entrust my very life to, not that I didn't do that with everyone else; so much so that most of the times I fall asleep during my morning routine. You know its trust when you have slept through a full bowel regimen: repositioning, numbing of your rectum, insertion of suppository and numerous digital stimulations; never waking until a warm washcloth touches your face after second repositioning.

In early 2016 I started having what we thought was respiratory problems that sometimes made it hard to swallow or breathe. I was wondering if my Sarcoidosis had worsened, up until now I hadn't shown symptoms. I was only diagnosed after having swollen lymph nodes appear on an ultrasound for something totally unrelated in 2004. I was admitted to UVA hospital for a battery of tests after a severe episode that left me trapped inside myself unable to communicate. I became ill, once again because of a kidney infection that worsened into sepsis. During 87% of my hospitalizations they have been because of kidney issues. When the inflamed nodes were detected I was having my abdomen scanned for kidney stones. If it can be produced by your body, mine will find a way; I have always been a medical abnormality. At that time in 2004 I was septic and hospitalized for 2 weeks. But back to more present times I had been back and forth to the emergency room 3 or more times with unfound problems. One morning after hiring a new attendant in February 2016 I was finishing breakfast and the last bite got stuck as I swallowed, I was scared because I couldn't cough it up, couldn't swallow it down or call for help. By the grace of GOD the attendant walked back in just in time and got my son to do a "Quad cough". Unfortunately, needless to say I scared an already timid person almost to death and she didn't return to work ever.

The last episode that eventually got me hospitalized on April 16th started more than a week before surgery. I'm sort of piecing this time together from other folk's memories because I have a very vague recollection of that period, so please bear with me. On or about the 6th I had another episode that got me hospitalized for a test because I was hurting and suspected another UTI, unaware of how ill I was; I got admitted with sepsis after a viral UTI for 6 days. I was discharged on the 12th just to sleep in my bed only 1 night and be readmitted for a worsening respiratory infection from the 13th through the 16th. Everyone around me was growing more concerned and frustrated because the hospital kept sending me home when it was apparent to my friends and family that something else was going on with me. The revolving door thing continued on Wednesday 18th when I was readmitted once again with respiratory failure, upper airway obstruction. Unresponsive when Ms. Peaches came into my room to get started that morning, after no usual good morning; Ms. Peaches realized something wasn't right and dialed 911. I was hospitalized for over a week while undergoing different tests and being treated for my diabetes which was severely elevated. My health issues since my paralysis can usually be categorized 1 of 3 ways: neurological, urological, or skeletal. I was once again septic because of a urinary tract infection but it was GOD's way of getting doctors to explore further and discover my bigger problem. Since my mental status was compromised also; it warranted a closer look. Being so ill I didn't even know what was going on, not exactly in a coma because I was still interacting with folks but I have no memory of that time (the lights were on but no one was home). Finally after a week and much poking, prodding, internal scanning, and family questioning; exams revealed abnormalities with my thyroid. My thyroidectomy was schedule for April 26/16 and I refused I've been told maybe subconsciously I knew I didn't want to go under the knife on the date that my mother died, terrified of surgery all my life a little senility didn't sway my protesting; Dr. Becker had to talk me into having life-saving surgery. Maybe I had a premonition or maybe it was GOD because the O.R. reserved for the 26th didn't get used that day because of a faulty O^2 plug. Maybe everything happened as it was meant to. My surgery was done on the 27th and because of complications due to infections I died twice on the operating table and after a second resuscitation slipped into a coma and doctors gave up on my full recovery. I was on a ventilator and comatose for at least a month. I was transferred to the transitional care (long term) hospital. I woke up somewhere after May 21, my dad's birthday.

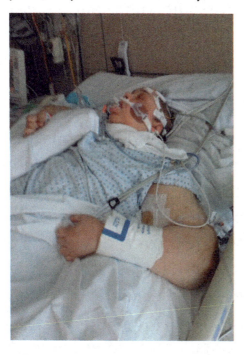

The human body is a wondrous piece of mystery… I don't know at what date or stage of my recovery I was in, when I had each dream, ongoing memory, or hallucination but I'm convinced that our bodies have a way of protecting us from things we can't handle, bringing us through and revealing truths in ways that God wants us to learn. It's been pointed out each time I became septic that I'm not in control; but it is okay because God is. I also believe that God uses our dreams to reveal things to us that we wouldn't or couldn't accept or understand while awake. I also believe that He use familiars to ease us through:

1. Good things: best friends, happy occasions and favorite color
2. Bad things: known enemies, sad or hard occurrences and dark colors.
3. Undetermined things: neutral people, never been to places and animals.

I think our unconscious mind can receive, process, and believe better and faster than our conscious mind. I also feel that God uses these familiars in conjunction with each other (antagonistically) as our yin and yang. I think our dreams are our subconscious directing our thought process. In my case every time I become septic I have vivid life projections. I can remember at least 3 times. About 12 years ago during a hospitalization for a urinary tract infection, one of those times I waited too long at home and lapsed into a semi- vegetative state for over a week. I can remember feeling as though I was strapped to a hospital bed, on trial between heaven and hell. I was being dangled almost upside down just being held to the bed by 4 point restraints. I remember people that were in my life at that time being asked whether I should be spared to live or should I die; if death is heaven or hell? As time went on that week it was revealed to me a few things:

1. That most people liked or loved me.

2. That I needed to remove some people from my inner circle.

3. That I needed to strengthen my faith or trust my higher power completely.

Each time thereafter when I was septic the revelations were to explain that I would be okay and to prepare me for upcoming events. The last time it happened made me aware that I needed to stop talking about writing this story, quit procrastinating and be about what I needed to do. The period between 4/1/2016- until the end of the year was spent in and out of the hospital, mostly because of the usual UTI's and respiratory issues. I don't remember much of that time because of encephalitis. I don't know much exactly about the day of my surgery except what I've been told. Dr. Becker told me after I woke up that they loss me twice during surgery. In order to successfully perform my surgery I had to be under major anesthesia. Because of it being throat surgery I ended up on a Ventilator. I was told that my family was informed that I would be Vent-Dependent the rest of my life; thankfully God had other plans. I was also made aware of just how alarmed everyone had been. I learned that I have protected my children too much throughout their life; so much so that they left everything about my care up to Peaches. Thank God for her and her support system through that period. I remained comatose for approximately 1 month after the beginning of this nightmare. I woke up around Memorial Day ravenous, but unable to eat solid food. I astonished the doctors and infer orated my speech pathologist because I wanted to resume eating anything I craved. I had to be staged back into solid food eating. I was only allowed pureed and soft foods. I wanted everything that I was accustomed to, bland baby food wasn't satisfying or filling. I was weaned from the ventilator by my birthday and really missing solid food and home. It was hard for me to accept that I shouldn't be eating whatever I wanted whenever I wanted until the time I encountered my first throat freeze while eating ice cream. It's a little daunting to swallow even melting ice cream and have it close off your throat temporarily. Still that wasn't enough to convince me I should be careful reintroducing my favorites, the right way; slowly. I found myself craving cheese popcorn one evening and because my son loves me, after working all day that Saturday. Demetrice stopped by a convenience store and brought a huge bag out to TCH, like big kids at a slumber party; we watched TV, giggled and devoured every cheesy salty melt in your mouth kernel. Still stubborn, determined and foolish I enjoyed that night sneaking popcorn until I almost choked when the salt made my throat spasm. I never revealed this to anyone until now. I had to get respiratory to suction my throat out earlier than scheduled that evening. I think I took my survival for granted until that moment. Looking back remembering how the suction catheter felt sliding into the hole in my throat, how the pressure built up as the tube slid into my upper larynx and how panicky I would feel if the tube felt like it went in too far into my lung. The sound of the mucus being sucked from my chest was worse than the slurping at the bottom of your favorite milkshake cup. The feeling was as if someone was trying to rip my lung out through a drinking straw. After I started behaving it was about a month until I was totally weaned from the ventilator and got the tube removed from my airway. I still needed to be suctioned in the mornings and sometimes after meals the first few days but by day 3 we had to use the cough assist machine only because the hole had closed completely. I knew I was on the road to healing. Wow another long journey almost over or so I thought. Again another UTI and some kind of infection I picked up in the hospital so another round of high dose antibiotics that had to be given intravenously so my discharge plans changed. Dr. Kevin Smith had filled in for the covering intern during the last month and took an interest in my case and thought some strengthening and re- training would be beneficial after discharge. He was now the go to spinal cord guru at Health-south's inpatient hospital so he asked if I'd like to come straight from T.C.H. I talked it over with Peaches because this would mean another two weeks without a paycheck. Yes she'd been by my side from April until then October 6th (my mom's birthday) without being paid or even sleeping in her bed at her house. When she did finally start leaving for the night which wasn't until I was totally off the ventilator and able to speak for myself... now, that's caring, dedication and love. Back to health-south my butt hit the bed an hour or so before dinnertime so nothing that night but registering. Unfortunately Friday we couldn't really do much either, because I didn't have my wheelchair, lift and clothing so Dr. Smith wasn't happy but said to work it out over the weekend we're hitting the ground running on Monday. Nine a.m. Dr. Smith and my physical therapist both came to do range of motion and discuss the care plan for my stay. During range of my right leg I grimaced so to be careful, informed about my abilities and the cause of the pain he ordered full body ex-rays and to our amazement discovered that my right femur was broken and sent me to orthopedic clinic and discharged me to UVA Hospital for surgery. Everything seems to happen on significant dates around my mom does this mean she's looking out for me or still has her fingers on my life from the grave. God stepped in again to turn it for me, thank God for keeping me yet again. I never checked into health-south anymore after I was discharged because I had to be very careful with that leg while it was healing. I still don't know if the box in my chest even works anymore or if it could be the source of my recurring infections.

Finally home for over a year, it's now black Friday 2018 and Peaches was tired of saying or hearing me say I didn't know my medical history because I was adopted. She gave me the ancestry.com kit for Christmas. I received it by mid-December but because of my own insecurities it set on my dresser for another month until almost February. My oldest son was here on January 24, 2019 when Peaches was leaving for the weekend, she grabbed it, slammed it in his chest and said make sure she does this before you leave. I knew I should have done it as soon as I got it but I have always been so scared that I would find out that my birth mom didn't want to find me or want me at all. So not searching didn't hurt me the way the truth could. Even though I had sent away years ago for the non-identifying information that revealed what I opened this book with, she was a teenage mother that struggled with her decision. I didn't want to upset her life. Also remembering the look on my adoptive mother's face some 45 years earlier as if I just screamed her inadequacies to the world. She had feared this very day since I became a permanent fixture in their lives. I remember being really angry with Barbara, my adoptive mom because I was struggling with foster placement, being very lonely and the separation from everything and everyone familiar was killing me. I couldn't call Willie because of her stupid idea that I actually left home to be able to be with him, I left because of her. When someone gives you 3 options you choose one and go with it. I chose option 3, to get the hell out of her house. Even though I knew it wasn't how I wanted to begin motherhood, but, I had to protect my unborn child and myself. The next morning after the frying pan attack still aching in my back from the blow, I knew for sure that her resentment of my pregnancy was growing and her love for me had charged into disgust. Her perfect daughter has become an evil woman she no longer could control. Her reputation is now tarnished by my unruliness. My desire for someone to love unconditionally and to love me the same threatened her hold on everyone in her inner circle. My father didn't approve of how I was being treated and he wouldn't ostracize me as she did. He was caught in the middle and refused to take her side, even though standing up to her wasn't in his nature, I recognized his supportive tone when he did speak. I hated the rift between us because my father was always the biggest cheerleader of my every endeavor. When I ran track he attended all the home meets and when we returned from away trips he was there waiting when the bus pulled in no matter the time. Every parade within 50 miles of Emporia he was at the finishing point to pick me up. Although he didn't have a high school education or even know how to read well he could build anything and there wasn't anything on God's green earth he wouldn't do within reason to provide my every whim. I've never known a more loving, loyal and well-tempered individual, unlike Barbara it took so much to anger him. I only once made him angry enough to give me a whipping and I truly believe it did hurt him more than me. I spoke out of turn and embarrassed him in W. T. Tiller hardware store in front of 3 white folks because I corrected a statement. Although the correction saved him money, my attempt to spin the situation eased their minds but one commented that he should make me his secretary, but it made him lose face or made him wonder if they knew that he couldn't read. After that incident he and I would work on reading every night for 2 years.

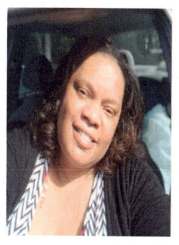

Sorry I got lost or off on another tangent and forgot what I was talking about. Well back to 2019, the test had been gone for just under three weeks and I got that email that made me jittery, scared and nervously anticipative; not only did I have a leaf but I had a message. Two days before Valentine's I found out that I have a younger sister on my mother's side that has known I existed all of her life. We definitely can't ever deny each other because just standing beside one another you definitely can tell we're related. Same complexion, same mannerisms, same body shape and even the same non existing eyebrows. Mommy wanted us to be able to find each other one way or the other. The only obvious differences are she's really the city mouse to my country mouse; whereas I'm a homebody she's the wanderer, traveling is her passion. I'm the only one with children and I don't think she wants any of her own. I also found out about a huge amount of family on my father's side but that doesn't matter so much to me. I finally have the one missing piece in my life, a sister. Already she's done that one thing that little sisters are good at... raiding my closet!

As Iyanna told me about our mother I found out that I was her doppelganger just as Demetrice is mine and his son his; I said all that to say the resemblance is undeniable. We look exactly alike at the same ages if you compare pictures of the same age of all 4 of us it's crazy. We even pursued the same line of work, nursing. The very year I wished for the love of my mother, any mother; my birth mother died doing her

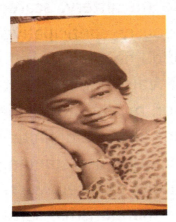

favorite activity, bowling. I learned that she had several heart attacks over a three year span because of a heart defect, courtesy of a drug addicted mom. She succumbed to that last one in a bowling alley in 1982, 53 days before my first child was born. Life can really deal some crazy blows sometimes right? The very things I feared for decades were farther from true as we were in distance. I also had it confirmed that she regretted having to give me up that she was forced by her grandma.

Made in the USA
Columbia, SC
03 July 2022